I0830050

Dedication

To my wife, Nandini, who encouraged me to continue when I wanted to give up, and shown me the deepest love.

To my sister, Nithya, who taught me to read and slogged through the first edits with me.

To my brother, Adithya, whose determination is a force to be reckoned with.

To my parents, who fought so hard to get us to where we are now.

Love you all.

Important Information for the Reader

The information presented in this book comes from my clinical experience and research from peer-reviewed studies. I offer my expertise to shed light on the relationship between diet, exercise, stress, and health. This book is neither for self-diagnosis or treatment of disease nor a substitute for the advice and care of a licensed health care provider. Sharing the information in this book with your attending physician is a great idea.

After reading this book, I can only hope that you make better judgments concerning your long-term health goals. If you are experiencing health problems, you should consult a qualified physician immediately. Remember, early examination and detection are essential to the successful treatment of all diseases.

Table of Contents

Introduction

To many people, this is a book about chiropractic. To some, this is a book about one person's fight for individuality and recognition. To a few, this is a book about hope and taking that proverbial leap of faith. I sincerely believe that telling my story is the means to a better understanding of my profession, and ultimately a better understanding of the idea of health.

I care deeply about what I do. I don't get up in the morning to go to work – I just get up and help people out. I'm a Chiropractor and damn proud of it. I don't have a magical fairy tale story on how I got into the profession. I was never a hardcore athlete who decided to become a Chiropractor after being miraculously fixed with treatment. I wasn't the latest in an extended family lineage of Chiropractors to join the field. Some of my colleagues were adjusted from birth, and some were patients with a chiropractor for most of their adult life. Not me, though.

The truth is, my first ever chiropractic treatment was in my first semester of Chiropractic College, that too by an intern (she was a genius, by the way)! This seemed incredible to my classmates. How could someone who a chiropractor had never treated want to become one? In fact, I didn't fully know either. I bet my first semester's tuition that this was a profession for me, based on the cursory research I had put into at that point.

The path to my first-ever chiropractic treatment was an excruciating process. The program at New York Chiropractic College was well planned. Being 1st-semester students, we paired with senior students in the clinical phase of their study, practicing in the student clinic. The student clinic was a set of treatment rooms assigned to clinical student interns under the watchful eye of a seasoned clinician and professor, typically from a technique course. First-year students were to schedule appointments with their interns based on their health requirements. The resulting win-win situation was that the intern could finally adjust patients and get the feel of being a clinician, and the freshman got free Chiropractic care. My first intern, God bless her soul, was extremely thorough. It took three agonizing appointments to get through the assessment. While all my classmates spoke about the treatments they had received, and bragged about the relief they were experiencing, I could only imagine what was in store.

Finally, the day came. My assessments were complete. I had no history of injury, and we waited for the sign-off from the supervising clinician. What was about to happen? What was going to change? Was it going to be painful? A whirlwind of thoughts and ideas flew through my head until I heard, "Okay, Prat. You ready?" In an instant, I was back in the treatment room, getting positioned for my adjustment. I kept thinking to myself, if I had no real issues, was this going to make a difference?

As I walked back to my dorm room after my session, a classmate passed me in the hall. I must have had a goofy grin on my face because she looked at me puzzled, with one raised eyebrow. "Are you okay?" She asked, genuinely curious. My instant response, without taking a second to think about it, "I've never been better." And I floated down the rest of the hallway back to my room. Nothing in that moment could have been more authentic. I genuinely felt the difference of having the restrictions in my spine corrected, and I felt a hundred pounds lighter. I felt relaxed. It was on that breezy evening, as I floated back to my dorm room smiling, I decided I had placed the right bet and that this was the profession for me. I would now spend my days giving people this immeasurably content feeling and be a beacon of hope for their pain and suffering.

The truth is, the spinal adjustments I had received were unlike any sensation I'd felt before, save for one instance in my childhood. That was a situation where my younger brother and I were fighting for the Intercontinental Championship, and he'd delivered a Macho Man Randy Savage elbow from the top rope as I lay on the carpet in the family room. Something didn't feel right, and my arm just wasn't able to be lifted past a certain level. It wasn't excruciating pain, but it definitely hurt. So, doing her diligence, Dr. Mom checked on me before bed. She rubbed my shoulder, and as she was squeezing it, she raised my arm. POP! No pain, complete movement. Slept like a baby.

My parents influenced my decision to become a doctor early. This wasn't a typical "Indian parent ideals" situation either, where the only three professions on earth were doctor, lawyer, or engineer. My father was a battler and fought through extreme odds to get our family started in Canada. From a tiny agricultural village in Andhra Pradesh, he excelled in his studies and eventually became a mechanical engineer with a decent job in Bangalore. He learned a great deal from growing up poor and conservatively planned his way to further career possibilities. He was selected for an exchange program to Germany through sheer determination and grit, where he would eventually meet my mother's two elder brothers.

Once again, his upbringing and hard-knock childhood allowed him to avoid common pitfalls that befell his colleagues. Being a young, Indian bachelor in the middle of Germany during the 70s, the temptations were numerous. My father's father had passed away at an early age due to an unfortunate snake bite. So, at the tender age of 10, my father became the man of the house, taking care of his mother and two younger siblings. He took classes during the day, and by evening tended the cows in the pasture or the groves of mango and coconut. That early responsibility held him in check through his time in Germany and allowed him to focus on his other goals.

After meeting my mother, and an arranged marriage later, he opted to shift to Canada through another opening from his German company. Less than 30 years of age, he moved to two different countries, got married, and bought a house. This was a man with a plan. My siblings and I owe him a lot in our ability to live a comfortable life. He overcame disproportionate odds and helped us succeed with nothing more than an iron will. He would not give up under any circumstances.

He had never leaned on any of us to become a doctor, lawyer, or engineer, but he was thoroughly disappointed when my sister decided against being a doctor when she was in the tenth grade. I'm sure that deep down, some part of my father had that dream of one of his children becoming a doctor, so this really took the wind out of his sails. Not very subtly, he'd drop hints about the economic benefits of being a doctor. I picked up on this vibe, and it framed my early ideas of what my future could be.

My own experience with doctors was not extremely pleasant. There were the stuffy offices. There were the stressful car rides from overly distressed parents. There were the allergy tests and antibiotics that were inevitably administered. Our family doctor seemed to love prescribing medicines, so much so that my siblings and I would often joke about which flavor antibiotic we'd get for our sore throat. I preferred banana. There were instances where he would not even check us but would busily prescribe antibiotics after a quick once over. He was a pleasant man, but I got the idea he wasn't terribly interested in our health.

After a routine visit to the dentist, and as we waited for my mother to finish her cleaning, my father shared the details of our family visit's bill. This was the first time I had ever been invited to look at anything related to finances, costs, or prices. I suppose my father decided that this was "The Time." It made an indelible impression. The numbers I was looking at were enormous, especially for 11-year-old me. His conclusion was simple – dentists make good money. Through numerous conversations over the next few years, my plan was easier to understand. I wouldn't have to go through the murky waters of being a medical doctor. No way was I going to sit back and prescribe my way through life. Dentists had a real thing going for themselves: they got to be doctors (check!), they made good money (check, check!), and they got to work with their hands (triple check!). And hey, as long as people had teeth, they'd need a good dentist. And so, it was settled; I was to become a dentist.

Mom hit me with a different set of ideas. She was your typical working-class supermom, working a day job, coming home, and handling household tasks. She was always sore. Her shoulders, her back, her neck. And so, when mom complained of a shoulder ache, I would dig my elbow into the stubborn knots. All the kids would take turns trying out their techniques to see who could help mom the most with her pain. Eventually, she just asked me. Sometimes after a session of elbow prodding, she would tell me her pain was all gone and that I had "healing hands."

She encouraged me to 'work' on her friends who would visit, nothing more than a motherly brag about a child's growing skill. "Meena, you should let Prathap press your shoulder. It instantly reduced my pain!" And sure enough, there I was, auntie by auntie, getting that small dose of experience related to muscles and the issues that plagued them.

As a sports enthusiast, I always took a keen interest in the players on my favorite teams and would follow the news about them avidly. In those days, the newspaper had a condensed segment for injuries on the last page of the sports section, and I would pore over the details for each league. Just by observation and repetition, I soon realized that when Kirk Muller came down with a knee sprain, he'd be out 2-4 weeks.

I was a good student, a decent athlete growing up, and a healthy level of self-confidence. It was easy to tell people I was going to be a dentist. I had dreamed of a future with a big house, picket fence, and Ferrari in the garage. Up to this point, things were easy, juggling all the pressures of being an outgoing teenager. Reality only hit like a ton of bricks once I entered university. I opted to test my independence and took my talents two and a half hours away from home to the University of Western Ontario.

As many college students realize, campus life is more about organization and structure than freedom. Sure, there's tons of space to explore, but only when armed with keenly sharpened time management skills. Young, cocky me bit off way more than I could chew, and after my first semester, I could feel the water rising with my head barely above it. After being a successful high school student, I was getting my first bitter taste of disappointment. What I didn't realize at the time was that *everybody* in university was *somebody* in their high school. It was a congregation of big dogs, and shit was about to get real. I made friends, people liked me, but it was different living away from home. I didn't know how ill-prepared I was to tackle the variety of challenges of on-campus life. After borrowing my friend's notes and comparing them to mine, I could see that some of my peers could handle this workload a lot better than me. I fell behind. I didn't do well.

During the summer vacations in university, I worked different jobs through a marketing company I had previously worked for as a teenager. The gigs were well paid, even if they had no relevance to my career path. In one of these instances, I first came across the idea of being a Chiropractor at all. Until this point, I had no concept of chiropractic other than they were a weird, "out there" type of health professional. Credit that to mainstream media perception. As I stood there on an endcap in a suburban Toronto Costco, demonstrating a particularly powerful vacuum that never ran out of suction, an attractive middle-aged woman walked by, to whom I decided to run my spiel.

"Need a new vacuum?" I asked with a smile as she was about to stride past. She slowed down, turned her head, then stopped. Over her shoulder, she asked, "why would you assume I do the vacuuming in my house?" I quickly changed course. "Does your husband need a new vacuum?" She turned around and walked up to my tiny demonstration station, literally a square of carpet and some tiny multicolored beads. "Okay, so why do I need this vacuum?" We joked and smiled through our conversation, and finally, she asked, "So what's your deal? Is this your full-time thing, or are you studying?" I told her that I was a Biology major and that I had plans to pursue dentistry. She smirked. "Dentistry, eh?" I looked her over. "I suppose you're some kind of Doctor?" I guessed correctly. She reached into her purse and pulled out a business card: Dr. Cecile Thackeray, Chiropractor. Dr. Cecile finished with a challenge: "You should come to my office; I'll give you ten reasons why Chiropractic is better than dentistry." I don't remember if she bought the vacuum or not. I didn't take her up on her offer, either.

The remainder of my university career was a roller coaster of achievement and personal growth. My self-esteem had taken a beating, and I had very slowly realized that my dreams of dental school were disappearing faster than Jell-O shooters at a sorority party. Some would argue that I just had to keep plugging away and have a singular focus to achieve the unlikely. My hope was fading, but still, I continued to pursue that goal. Either way, I had come far, through some teeth clenching, gallons of coffee, and virtually living at the library. I clinched the dramatic turnaround in my final year by earning a spot on the Dean's List. It was during that pivotal 4th year that my friend Benjamin Bluestein threw an idea at me. "Why don't you apply for Chiropractic College?"

I rejected the idea outright. Chiropractic? Coincidentally, Ben had similar plans for his postgraduate study. Like me, he had designs on becoming a dentist. But he planted the earworm successfully. It tunneled, grew, and took hold deep in there. Also, coincidentally, he is now a practicing Chiropractor in Hong Kong. You can't make these things up.

I looked up programs in Canada and was astonished that only two programs were available in the whole country. I looked south of the border and found tons more. New York Chiropractic College stood out, and I started the process of applying to the program because, as Ben correctly pointed out, you never really know.

I sent in my transcripts and my interest letter, then very quickly had a telephone interview set up with Dr. Thomas Ventimiglia, a professor at NYCC and veteran chiropractor. It was a genuinely pleasant conversation, more like warm acquaintances greeting each other after a long gap in their conversation. He asked about my family and my current situation. He asked about my experience with chiropractic. Dr. Ventimiglia was as baffled as my future classmates about how I could consider applying to a program with zero personal experience. He concluded our conversation with some actionable steps to understand the program and the profession better. After I agreed to shadow a Chiropractor for a few weeks, he signed off by saying, "Okay! The game is afoot!" I'll never forget that conversation.

A week later, I was issued a conditional acceptance from NYCC, contingent upon my volunteer work with a licensed Chiropractor. However, after a long chat with my folks, I opted to defer my admission to continue pursuing dentistry.

Here's where I hit fast forward. Upon graduating from Western with a BSc in Honors Biology, I applied to multiple dental programs and, unfortunately, was denied admission to all of them. My dreadful first-year grades continued to hold me back, and the various professional departments had mixed opinions about my chances of being admitted. I continued to do a year of undergraduate studies at York University, closer to home, and with coursework 'out of my concentrated area of expertise' in order 'to diversify my transcript.' Whatever that meant. With a better grade point average, I applied again, more schools this time around, more applications, but still came up empty. Zilch. Nada. Bupkis. Not wanting to pursue a Master's degree or ship out to the Caribbean or dental schools overseas, I found a job as a surgical assistant at a leading laser eye surgery company. It was here that I finally started looking at other avenues of study, however, to no avail. Optometry, Audiology, and Physiotherapy were all highly competitive programs, but for me, just a row of closed doors. Nobody wanted me, as it turned out.

With dwindling options, I decided to reach out to New York Chiropractic College once more. My thought process was simple - they wanted me once, why not again, two years later? So, with my back up against the wall, I asked about reactivating my admission. Thank goodness for not-so-small mercies. They accepted my request and fast-tracked my admission process while I updated my references. Bada boom, bada bing. Now I just had to convince my folks about this life-altering decision. No pressure, right?

Two years before, when I'd told my folks about being accepted to NYCC, they met this idea with all kinds of skepticism. Dad was very vocal about having 'singular focus' and 'not getting distracted from your goal.' Mom was apprehensive about the validity of chiropractic. Neither of them had much confidence in it, and both had summarily written the profession off as a general unknown. This time, I pitched the idea softly. Their initial wariness on this turned to a sort of relief. They were happy that I would be entering into a doctoral-level program. They were delighted I had decided. There were some concerns about moving to the U.S., finances, and other procedural and logistical doubts. But ultimately, with their blessing, I took the plunge and hit accept on the offer of admission.

I honestly believe, whatever forces compelled me or steered my decision-making, I made the right decisions at the right time. Kismet, if you will. I could not imagine doing anything other than what I'm doing now. The ability to change lives, in some cases, almost immediately, is nothing short of a gift. I cherish my responsibility as a healthcare provider, and I try to impact everybody's life I touch positively. I am keenly interested in my patients' lives; restoring not just movement to a joint but putting more *life* into their lifestyle is a fantastic feeling. It's hard to put into words, but this, in a nutshell, is *why* I do what I do.

Chiropractic remains a poorly understood profession. When I was first introduced to it many years ago, I was skeptical. The same was true when I brought the idea to my parents for the first time. Their gut reaction was just fear of the unknown. It seems that just the name alone raises many questions, let alone about the origins of chiropractic, how to use it, and how it is accepted by the mainstream medical field today. That is one of the purposes of this book.

Another reason I wanted to write a book on chiropractic was to give both my patients and chiropractic skeptics a look at the logic behind this science. Yes, despite what exists out there on the interweb, chiropractic is a science, is professionally researched, and has scientific evidence to prove its effectiveness. As more medical doctors and other health professionals realize the benefits of proper chiropractic care, the number of inter-professional referrals is also increasing. Patients they once thought could only be treated by prescription drugs and surgery are now being trusted into the non-invasive, gentle care of their local chiropractor.

Putting this book together, I turned to the go-to strategy that I use in my practice – teamwork. I sought out the experience of other chiropractors to add their expertise, research, and insights to my own in creating a well-rounded publication. I want to inform and educate my readers on chiropractic and how to live a life centered on wellness and hopefully re-illustrate the whole idea of health. Tons of Chiropractors have written books about chiropractic, and I add my name to that list. I hope to accomplish, where others have failed, a simple, easy-to-read overview of the profession and how it works. I also offer you a piece of myself, as I provide instances and examples of my own experiences, trials, and triumphs. I want my audience to feel included in this journey without alienating them, using technical jargon and industry slang.

This gave great purpose to my publication. I wanted a sensible summary of various medical conditions and lifestyle choices that can help you better understand the basics of how chiropractic can help improve your way of life.

This book's more extensive scope is to educate and inform readers about the part chiropractic plays specifically regarding best practices in mental health, physical health, and the role of wellness. Wellness is the idea of harmony and balance for all aspects of your life. This book considers that chiropractic with other lifestyle choices and good habits can create a sense of wellness beyond fighting disease and illness.

Good health and high spirits go hand in hand. Understanding how each activity you participate in relates to all other lifestyle factors is crucial to achieving even the most minor health goals. Being "well" in every sense of the word connects every step you take to feed and nourish your body and mind and how you react to external factors.

Finally, my number one reason for writing this book is to empower the reader to take steps they may have been reluctant to take to improve their health, connect to their world around them, and refine their lifestyle. There's no point in just plugging in and living on autopilot. I wish to share with you, not teach, not preach. I want you to arrive at your own conclusions, as I hope to alleviate fear and shed some light on the unknowns surrounding chiropractic. I want everybody reading this book to embrace a preventative maintenance lifestyle that encourages freedom from stress, pain, and suffering.

So, what can you expect from this book? Common sense! As a culture, we inundate our minds with thinking that for something to work, it has to be complicated. Nothing could be further from the truth. If it's complicated, people won't use it. It's that simple.

The technology space is an excellent example of an industry that is revolutionizing through simplicity. Think about it! A website used to take weeks to code and launch. With the technology currently available, this might only take hours. This growing sector of technology only exists to make things easier. The health industry is due for a learning revolution by creating concepts that are easy to understand. The easier the idea, the more it is used in reality. If it's not simple, you will have all the excuses in the world not to use them.

We'll be talking about the body, health conditions, as well as things that are simple to do that can make a huge difference in your overall health. Goals must look doable, or we aren't even going to attempt them. Step by easy step, we'll break down each challenge you may face in creating a world of difference in your life.

People often say that patience is a virtue. What the heck does that even mean? The Oxford dictionary defines virtue as "behavior showing high moral standard." In our case, I'm going to change this idea slightly. Instead of patience being the behavior of high *moral* standards, we will regard it as the behavior of high *functional* standards. We always believe that we can change our lives overnight. The truth is that we can change our *mind* overnight, but our body doesn't change that quickly. Patience is required to aid our transition and function to help us achieve the desired change.

Let's say we have chronic low back pain. Most people look at the *last* thing that happened before they started to feel the pain. The truth is, whatever it was that created the condition of our body, didn't build up over the last one or two weeks and certainly didn't happen overnight; it took a lifetime. All the decisions and choices you made to this point in your life can and will factor into your body. So, if you want to change your health for the better, you must look at the element of patience differently. Look at it as an ongoing process that you begin today. Use this book as a compass and keep guiding yourself towards a better life.

All you need to do to get value out of this book is to begin by opening your mind and being receptive. People say the mind is like a parachute, and it won't work if it's not opened. You must have an open mind to receive new ideas to be put into action. Most people are not well. Some element of their life is facing challenges they are unable to overcome. Simplicity, patience, and an open mind are the recipe for change, especially for actions that the mainstream population may not commonly use.

We, as a society, fear change. Yet, we continue to march on the path that has brought us to our current experience of health, despite how much better it could be if we embraced change. Somehow, in our minds, we expect that staying on the same path can yield different results than the last time we started down it. This is terribly similar to a popular definition of insanity – doing the same thing repeatedly, expecting different results. Curiosity might be the catalyst you need to bridge the gap from where you are to where you want to be. Be curious about things; try new stuff! Don't have tunnel vision. Be open to new possibilities. Be patient in trying something new and be prepared to find it not "working at first," after all, it took your whole life to get you to where you are now.

Interestingly, society believes that we must succeed on the first attempt to be successful at something. This is a myth; it simply doesn't happen that way. The truth is that we learn through failure. Someone who never fails loses out on experience and the opportunity for growth. The slap that we feel from failing at something is a potent reminder not to approach the problem with the same solution but to be flexible, and change our thinking, even just a little bit. If success on the first attempt was the expected standard, babies would never need to crawl and never fall when they started walking. If a baby fell while trying to walk, would they sit there and think, "nope, that's it for me. I guess I'm not the walking kind?" This example is a bit silly, but as adults, we have this expectation. Let that sink in.

Life is a process. It is an experience. We must go through life with the courage that we will sometimes fall or sometimes fail. But, so what! All we do is just get back up. There are hundreds of sayings and idioms that come to mind describing this precisely. As this recipe for success grows increasingly longer, remember that simplicity is the main ingredient. An open mind is the mixing bowl. Patience is the functional measuring cup. And now perseverance is the whisk. Go whip up something good! Open your heart and open your mind and begin to explore the possibilities of a new life. The life I am talking about is a life with more energy, vitality, and most of all, a life full of HEALTH!

Chapter 1

Stumbling Blocks to Success

Fear is one of the biggest obstacles that can prevent you from getting anything from this book. Fear deprives you of desire and justifies why you continue to achieve substandard results. Don't let fear hold you back. It can rob you of your dreams, and it can indeed drain you of your health and well-being.

Excuses will dry up your motivation for change more than anything out there. Don't make any more excuses. 'Easier said than done,' I'll openly admit that. However, there is a saying, "If you can complain about it, you can do something about it. If you can't do something about it, no point in complaining." Don't let excuses be a barrier for you to implement what you learn from this book. Grab some strategies and go with them confidently. They say that it takes 21 days of consistency to create a good, healthy habit. This isn't a self-help book; it means to be a guide on making simple changes in your daily routine. It doesn't have to be complicated, and we're not trying to reinvent the wheel. Tiny drops at a steady rate will fill a bucket.

Many patients tell me, "I'm tired of feeling this; I don't want to feel pain anymore." Or they may say to me, "I don't want to feel tired anymore." They tell me what they *don't* want to feel. Many people are in this exact position. This moment is where I typically explain their primary barrier to success: they're setting themselves up to fail. The mind is powerful, and with that type of tunnel vision, "pain, pain, pain, ouch, ouch, oof," it quickly fails to see the way out. If all Susan thought about was what she didn't want to feel, how could she suddenly concentrate on what she *did* want? The mind starts to respond to and even give in to the negativity. It's a slippery slope, but thankfully, it is possible to self-correct with the proper guidance and suggestions. So, focus on what you want, not on what you don't want. It's not so much that you don't want to feel pain; it's more like you want to be able to play with your kids or get in a great round of golf! That mind shift is the key!

I hope that by reading this book, you too can decide that chiropractic care is a part of a health care and wellness routine that everyone needs -- not just those with back problems. It can provide you with a proactive approach to your health. It can also open the body up to its full self-healing potential. Not too many doctors and pharmacists would dare make that claim. I invite you to read on and learn more about this proven scientific method of wellness, and all that chiropractic encompasses.

The Simplicity Philosophy

Simplicity is a philosophy that a person can adopt for a lifetime. No, you don't need to trade in your suit and tie for traditional homespun and sit under a tree, either. You should grab onto things that can work. And guess what? Simple plans work. Excellent results await you as you read ahead. All you need is the confidence in yourself to implement the following information. Then you will find yourself making huge gains within your health. Neither was Rome built in a day, nor will optimal health. The ticket to that result? Consistently applied simple changes.

Remarkable healing powers are within you, waiting to unleash. The main point is to focus on the wins and not get distracted by the inevitable setbacks. Picturing yourself with what you desire – the big win – is what will take you over the hump, no matter the hurdles you'll face.

All of the principles you are going to learn in this book come from the laws of nature. They are not some magical, fad-like approaches that contradict simple common sense. They are simply truths that exist in the natural world around us, applied to different situations we may encounter. When we look at the grand design and the framework within which we all exist, you will notice the most basic details that make the miracle happen, and we're all the better for it. Healthy people are happy people, and happy people are better, more productive members of society.

The laws of nature are the same principles by which farmers abide. "Taking the bull by the horns," for example. This idea compels action; control the things around you rather than let what happens control your destiny. Many theories have substantial merit, but what good are they if you don't act upon them and are not consistent with your action?

One example is the yo-yo weight loss and gains cycle, which results from diet fads popularized from all corners of social media. You starve yourself for two weeks, and ta-da! You lost five pounds!

Yet three days later, several slices of pizza and cake later, you are right back where you started, sometimes even worse. Trying to do too much too soon, expecting miracles out of the box, and not being consistent are all typical outcomes of these "action plans." Health is not a destination or a finish line to cross. We can't perform a few actions, "arrive," and then fall off the wagon. Health is a moving target, and we must continuously pursue it!

Technology's Role in Health Care

Sure, technology has had a significant impact on healthcare. The invention of the x-ray and ultrasound allows us to see into the body and observe what we could only approximate before. Further advances in science and technology are only a hop, skip, and a jump away from creating a whole other reality in health. Hello, artificial intelligence! While that all sounds like it could be in a leading science-fiction title, the focus of this book is simplicity, a de-evolution from technology. We should not complicate health. Typically speaking, we want the experts to tell us what our problem is, label it, and give us hope that we can fix whatever ails us. It's at this critical moment that we forget our elementary intelligence, our common sense. It's also at this point that some health experts gobble you up, complicating matters, forcing you into a sort of a rabbit hole of dependency.

That has been the problem within certain medical professions for some time. We have abided by the opinions of our healthcare professionals and their latest technologies, but it has brought us no more health than we expected. According to the World Health

Organization (WHO), so-called "modern societies" like the United States fail miserably as a society regarding health. The WHO reports that the U.S. ranks 37th out of 200 countries in terms of quality of individual health and wellness, despite spending more dollars on healthcare. To put that into perspective, Colombia is ranked 39th.

The example of the USA is followed elsewhere in the world, too. What we are doing is simply not working. Innovation is at the heart of this book. No more complex strategies; we will get to the straightforward, bare-bones concepts that you can use immediately every day, and that can genuinely make a difference in your life.

Break away from the old and decide today for yourself to use a technology that will truthfully make a difference in your life. You deserve it, and those around you deserve someone who comes to the table alive, refreshed, energetic, and not just a partial representation of themselves. You deserve to reach the full you at your highest potential! It should not be an option or a fantasy; it should be your mission.

Why do we need to think outside the box? Like in my parents' example, there are more options than we allow ourselves to consider, more angles for solving problems. Our current paradigm is disease care – only once something breaks is when we think to fix it. The better way is preventative care – improve or keep up things *before* they break. It's the most cost-effective way of taking care of our bodies.

This preventative model is not a new concept in other trades, so why should it be so under-utilized regarding health? Automotive companies have known about it since the invention of cars. They are well aware that if you give your vehicle preventative care such as periodic tune-ups and oil changes, they will last longer. Dentists have it figured out as well, for a more relevant healthcare example. If you don't brush your teeth today, you won't immediately have a cavity tomorrow, but if you continue to neglect your oral hygiene, you most certainly will. The basic principle your dentist pounds into your head is that a simple check-up can prevent all those bad things, just twice a year. Oh, and floss. Definitely floss. It's that simple.

A big step forward is to trim the fat from our health care. I believe the best way to do that is not to rely on symptoms. Symptoms are usually an SOS from your body, letting you know that something needs attention. If you wait until there are symptoms, most often, you are too late. You will learn more about this later in the book, but please keep that concept in mind.

The tests and processes we are using to determine health are not showing the consequences of our diets of ten years ago. It doesn't show what will happen with our arteries 5 or 10 years from now if we continue eating the way we are. Healthcare costs will skyrocket if we carry on at this rate, creating a very scary "health-pocalypse." Even though health insurance costs aren't prevalent in every corner of the globe, the trend around the world shows alarming spikes in the prices of these services. Again, to use statistics from the U.S., healthcare costs are among the top reasons people file for bankruptcy. You can do your part to change this; we all can. All it takes is a slight change in our perception, where we approach our health in a preventative, proactive manner.

Chapter 2

The History of Chiropractic

Chiropractic is not a new idea. It is quite the contrary. In anatomy and physiology, the earliest physicians recognized the prominent role the spine played in health. Modern chiropractic fundamentally aims to facilitate the body to heal itself, in addition to promoting and maintaining wellness. Chiropractic claimed its first historic breakthrough in the late 19th century. It is incredible to think that was only a little over 120 years ago.

As with ancient Chinese herbal medicine, acupuncture, Ayurveda, or other "alternative medicines," chiropractic is considered holistic or non-allopathic. Chiropractic has a place in healthcare for those looking toward finding the cause of their pains and illnesses and treating them at the source instead of covering up symptoms with a temporary pain killer. Despite sharing the non-allopathic title with these other methods, chiropractic is a relative newcomer. For example, the practice of acupuncture dates back *thousands* of years. The history of chiropractic is still being written, as modern technologies blend with time-proven procedures to promote wellness.

Ancient History

Chinese and Greek writings dating back to 2700 BC imply that these ancient civilizations recognized the spine's role in health. The renowned Greek physician Hippocrates said, "Get knowledge of the spine, for this is the requisite for many diseases." Hippocrates wrote extensively about the spine. His recommended treatment for curvature of the spine, for example, stated:

"But the physicians, or some person who is strong, and not uninstructed, should apply the palm of one hand to the hump, and then, having laid the other hand upon the former, he should make pressure, attending whether this force should be applied directly downward, or toward the head, or toward the hips. This method of applying force is particularly safe." (Internet Classics Archive, 2021).

Hippocrates noted throughout his writings that the physician should be knowledgeable of the spine. He remarks on procedures that worked and mechanisms that did not work so well. This exploration of the body gave physicians and other types of non-traditional healers a foundation from which to build. They discovered how nerves, carefully protected by the bony structure known as the vertebrae or spinal column, could be critical in how the body took care of itself.

Chiropractic, once referred to as "bone setting," continued to be practiced for centuries until the fall of the Roman Empire. Much of the learning and medical practices were lost during this dark period in history. Fortunately, some techniques were not lost and got handed down from one generation to the next. Variations of "bone setting" were used throughout Europe and Asia during the 11th and 15th centuries. Another popular method that gained traction during this time - "back walking" - was the act of walking on someone's back to cure specific ailments and is still widely practiced in Southeast Asian countries.

By the 1800s, a period of "enlightenment" was occurring in Europe. Medical practitioners tried new procedures with some success. Indeed, "western" medicine had started its meteoric rise by vanquishing illnesses at surprising rates. These advances, however, made medical doctors shun bone setting, regarding it as an old-fashioned and ineffective method of treatment. There was one famous surgeon who held onto the merit of bone setting. In 1867, Sir James Paget gave credibility to spinal manipulation as a viable treatment in his article in the <u>British Medical Journal</u> entitled *Cases That Bone Setting Cures*. Unfortunately, the number of renowned medical doctors who supported the case for continuing spinal manipulation decreased drastically during this period.

The DD. Palmer Story

The story of "modern" chiropractic begins in 1895 with a man practicing as a magnetic healer. Daniel David (D.D.) Palmer lived and practiced in Davenport, Iowa. As a magnetic healer, he already recognized more options for treating a person than prescribing medicines. Magnetic healers felt a core of energy existed within a person that could help heal disease and keep people well. They realized that human beings possessed the right makeup and tools to heal themselves if whatever invasive element preventing optimum health was fixed or eliminated from the body.

One day, while in his office building, Dr. Palmer noticed that a janitor, a black man named Harvey Lillard, was almost entirely deaf. He asked the man how he lost his hearing. Lillard unfolded a story that would change Palmer's concept of healing forever and introduce chiropractic as a legitimate alternative means of health care. As Mr. Lillard's story progressed, he related an incident that happened some seventeen years earlier. He recounted that he felt a popping sensation in his neck or upper back while bending over. From that point forward, his hearing significantly diminished.

Dr. Palmer asked to examine Mr. Lillard, and upon touching the area he described, Dr. Palmer felt a large bump, which Mr. Lillard confirmed had been there ever since the incident. Dr. Palmer used his knowledge of anatomy to explain that it appeared that a vertebra had been displaced. With Mr. Lillard's consent, Dr. Palmer began to push on the bone, realigning it into its proper position.

The result was that Harvey Lillard regained his hearing. The proposed idea of this miracle was simple - the misaligned vertebra had been blocking the nerves' signals, putting pressure on the auditory sensors so that hearing was impaired. No one is sure whether it took several minor manipulations or if Lillard's hearing improved all at once. Within two years after the episode with Mr. Lillard, D.D. Palmer left the practice of magnetic healing and began working as a professional chiropractor.

The first school of chiropractic began in Davenport, Iowa, where Dr. Palmer was working. As it became known, the Palmer School of Chiropractic continued to grow as Dr. B.J. Palmer, D.D.'s son, continued in the family profession. This school is still in operation today as a renowned college of chiropractic. B.J. is given credit for increasing recognition and acceptance of chiropractic well into the 20th century.

Chiropractic as a profession faced opposition from the outset. Once the first graduating students of the Palmer School tried opening practices, they were troubled by the law. Without a license, authorities accused the new grads of practicing medicine illegally. Even Dr. D.D. Palmer stood accused, eventually serving a 23-day jail sentence and forking over $350 in fines. The act of jailing chiropractors for working with patients came to an abrupt halt due to a landmark case in Wisconsin. Dr. Shegataro Morikubo was acquitted because the judge and jury determined that he was not practicing medicine but performing a different type of healing, namely chiropractic. The law decided at the time that no license was required. Today, licensing is required of professional chiropractors by many different state and local regulatory agencies, along with rigorous nationalized board examinations.

What Does "Chiropractic" Mean?

The American Heritage Dictionary defines chiropractic (chi·ro·prac·tic) (noun) as:

"A system of therapy in which disease is considered the result of abnormal function of the nervous system. The method of treatment usually involves (the) manipulation of the spinal column and other body structures."

Its word root is Greek, from the words "cheiros," meaning "hand" and "praktos," which means "done by." In short, it is *the practice of using the hands*.

Professional organizations and groups governing the practice of chiropractic further expanded this definition in the following years. For example, the Massachusetts General Laws, Chapter 112, Section 89, describes chiropractic as:

"The science of locating and removing interference with the transmission or the expression of nerve force in the human body, by the correction of misalignments or subluxations of the bony articulations and adjacent structures, more especially those of the vertebra column and pelvis, for the purpose of restoring and maintaining health. X-ray and analytical instruments may be used for the purposes of chiropractic examinations."

Whereas the American Chiropractic Association (ACA) states:

"Chiropractic is a health care profession that focuses on disorders of the musculoskeletal system and the nervous system, and the effects of these disorders on general health. These disorders include, but are not limited to: back pain, neck pain, pain in the joints of the arms or legs, and headaches. Doctors of chiropractic (D.C.s) practice a conservative approach to health care that includes patient examination, diagnosis and treatment. D.C.s have broad diagnostic skills and are also trained to recommend therapeutic and rehabilitative exercises, as well as to provide nutritional, lifestyle and dietary counseling."

The common thread between these three different definitions of chiropractic is the nervous system. In the most specific version, the Massachusetts definition shows a focus on removing interference from nerve function. The ACA version is more generally worded and does not explicitly label the anatomy on which chiropractors must focus. Slight variations in context show diversity within chiropractic, leading to a spectrum of 'styles' incorporated in the profession. Within the group of practitioners that focus on wellness, it does not matter whether misalignment of the spine is due to injury or just natural changes that happen to the spinal column through everyday living. The idea is that by diligently checking and removing the interference, the opportunity for optimum health is there.

As some of you already know and others will discover, there are many different philosophies and practices throughout the chiropractic profession. Some chiropractors include much more than the adjustment of the spine in their approach. Since chiropractic is also considered a lifestyle modification, many other practices go along with spinal manipulations. Together, these take into account all aspects of wellness.

My chiropractic philosophy includes a combination of theories spanning generations and opposing viewpoints. The early versions of chiropractic hung on specific ideas based on theoretical or deductive science. This wobbly premise gave the medical community ample ammunition to dismiss chiropractic as "unscientific" summarily. The more modern versions of chiropractic rely heavily on scientific research, which doesn't always explain why some outcomes occur due to chiropractic care. I will always be identified or labeled as a 'mixer' within chiropractic communities. I cannot wholly embrace ancient dogma as scientific evidence, and I cannot dismiss the effect of thousands of chiropractors making changes to everyday people's issues, despite a lack of peer-reviewed, double-blind scientific literature for that specific problem.

Primarily, I look at the biomechanical issues a patient is facing first. I will factor in any possibility that a nerve, which controls the area of concern, is hindered in its function. I will then try to recreate the patient's bio-psycho-social environment to understand any additional contributors to their issue. I passionately believe that there are solutions to almost every problem a patient can face, and part of our job is to pull out our deerstalker hat à la Sherlock Holmes, and piece together the clues our patients give us. Chiropractors treat the body as a whole, which means figuring out a person's issue from a physical, chemical, and emotional level.

A Timeline of Chiropractic Development and Growth

Like anything medicine or healing-related, chiropractic has undergone growth and development over the last century. Modern technological advances in X-rays and other radiological scans have played a part in developing the scope of chiropractic. Each decade has brought exciting new advancements in understanding and acceptance among the public and how people manage their health care. Here is a timeline of highlights in the growth and knowledge of chiropractic:

385 BCE: First mention of spinal manipulation to treat back pain by Hippocrates. The details provided in this record suggest spinal manipulation was widely used and established as a practice by this time.

460 BCE: Hippocrates writes about the nervous system, joints, and manipulation.

195 CE: The correlation between healing and the nervous system, providing evidence for spinal manipulation, is discovered by Roman surgeon Claudius Galen.

1000-1674 CE: Prominent doctors (Avicenna, *The Book of Healing,* Friar Thomas, *The Complete Bone Setter,* Johannes Scultetus, *The Surgeon's Storehouse*) used and described manipulative methods identified by Hippocrates.

1800 onwards: Bone setters functioned in rural villages all across Europe and Asia after medicine becomes the favored practice in urban settings.

1887: D.D. Palmer opens the Palmer Infirmary of Magnetic Healing.

1895: D.D. Palmer helps restore the hearing of Harvey Lillard, a janitor who seventeen years earlier lost his hearing when he "heard a pop" in his upper back.

1897: The Palmer School of Magnetic Healing (later changed to the Palmer School of Chiropractic), the first college of its type, opens in Davenport, Iowa.

1902: Commencement held for the first graduating class of the Palmer School of Magnetic Healing. There were 15 graduates.

1904: Palmer school of Magnetic Healing officially changes its name to the Palmer School of Chiropractic.

1907: Lawsuit against Shegataro Morikubo for practicing medicine without license rules that he was practicing chiropractic, which at the time did not require licensure, and charges were dismissed.

1913: Kansas becomes the first state to license chiropractors.

1924: B.J. Palmer, D.D.'s son, starts the first radio station ever to be established west of the Mississippi in Des Moines, Iowa, and coins the term "broadcast." His station is called "WOC" for Wonders of Chiropractic.

1927: Chiropractic is now a licensed profession in 39 states.

1928: B.J. Palmer buys and airs the program termed "WHO" (With Hands Only), where he discusses his chiropractic experiences and travels.

1941: The first criterion for accrediting chiropractic colleges is established by John Nugent, DC, and starts the accreditation of 12 schools of chiropractic.

The Growth of Chiropractic Today

Chiropractic, as a fundamental practice, has not changed much in its 125 years of modern usage. It has only grown in popularity and acceptance. The same principles behind chiropractic remain unchanged. That fundamental understanding that the body is capable of self-healing controlled by the nervous system, and that this system regulates and operates every other organ and function within the body is the same today as in the past.

Currently, there are 46 officially, internationally accredited colleges of chiropractic in the world, spanning 19 different countries. The World Federation of Chiropractic (WFC) estimates over 100,000 chiropractors practice worldwide in over 90 countries. Chiropractors are the most numerous primary care professionals in the USA today, second only to medical doctors. The interest in the profession is growing, and with the latest failures from the mainstream medical model in the spotlight, natural holistic healing has once again become normal and widely accepted.

There has always been and will always be a strong relationship between the spine and wellness. If there is something out of order with the spine, it can lead to other health problems. Correct the problem with movement or alignment in the spinal column, and you open the body's ability to heal and correct that problem.

Chapter 3

What Is "Health?"

Suppose that I was to ask you to define the term "health." What kind of answer would you give me? There is a general opinion and consensus that good health is (1) feeling "fine," or (2) when everything is working okay, or (3) when pain or disease is absent.

All of these definitions are partial and independently are far from complete. Taber's medical dictionary defines health as "a condition in which all functions of the body and mind are normally active." The World Health Organization defines health as "a state of complete physical, mental or social well-being and not merely the absence of disease or infirmity." So, the next question to ask is, how does one quantify health?

In a sense, health is equal to balance. But how do you determine this balance? What are the determining factors in the balancing equation? To answer this, we must first ask, what are the elements to consider while determining health? Also, how do we measure the quality of health we experience?

To get to the core of good health, you need to start at the cellular level. The balancing act begins there. The quality of your life is based on the quality of the life of your cells. Since your body is composed of over 70 trillion cells, you can assume that you will have good health when those cells work in perfect harmony. But again, how does one quantify this?

Well, if health equals balance, we can think of it in terms of ease. Think of something or someone that is balanced. It's easy! There's no pressure pushing in any direction, or if there is, it doesn't show. We can then picture that the opposite of health is the opposite of ease. A state of "dis-ease" then refers to things being anything but balanced, kind of chaotic, and fighting to attain this equilibrium. In milder cases of this imbalance, we can say that the cells are not functioning correctly. Notice the difference between dis-ease and disease. Disease suggests suffering, pain, or even death. You can also say that 'disease' is an extreme form of dis-ease. Dis-ease refers to imbalance and may not even create pain or suffering.

Through his research, Raymond Francis, a chemist, bestselling author, and graduate of MIT, believes that only one thing creates disease. That reason is simply due to cells not functioning correctly. When you think about that statement, it makes sense. There are two primary reasons why cells do not perform well:

Cells are not receiving proper nutrition

Cells are not eliminating the toxicity produced by the normal functioning of the cell.

Secondary possibilities on what might make cells dysfunctional:

Lack of appropriate levels of oxygen

Improper nerve impulse to the cell

To begin to understand this process, let us quickly visit the stages of health. From conception onwards, we are born with the ability to develop healthily, effortlessly. However, suppose the intimate relationship between the nervous system and the rest of the body is disturbed. In that case, you will lose your efficient ability to develop, and therefore be healthy.

Initially, we only experience the effects of aging through a microscopic inspection. Long before we feel the effects of age, our cells begin to experience changes. Except for a few types, constant cell cycling allows for more efficient function. Through life, the process of cell production and elimination keeps the fittest, healthiest cells in living tissue. Once the cells begin to replicate less efficiently, it signals a transition from the anabolic stage of life (building) to a phase of catabolic metabolism. The catabolic stage marks a time that we have more cells that are dying than are being replaced. When we enter this point, we must do everything within our power to slow down the process.

Cells make up tissues. Tissues make up organs, muscles, and blood vessels. The combined effort of the organs, muscles, and blood vessels gives us life. It's no wonder then that cells are called the building blocks of life! When cells are in perfect balance (at ease, in good health), it has a particular term - *homeostasis*. This state signifies our optimal health where everything is working as designed.

However, as we age, we begin to encounter stresses in our lives, which signal cellular changes to the point where we will enter a phase of imbalance, lack of ease, or dis-ease. Stresses are either *physical*, *chemical*, or *emotional* in origin. One can quickly regain health if one can reduce stress and counter it with logical measures. Despite the aging process being inevitable and ubiquitous, there are measures we're all capable of to limit the damaging effects and still keep our lives in balance.

Varying levels of pain can accompany the initial cellular imbalances we experience, but not in all cases. Sometimes, there are no visible or sensed symptoms. If we stay in this phase for any actual amount of time, we begin to have dis-ease in more than one cell. It begins to affect thousands and thousands of cells to the point of reaching the body's tissue level. Left further without a reversal of the dis-ease, it enters into a larger group of tissues, affecting organs. It then moves onto systems, and then ultimately, it affects the entire being, which eventually leads to death.

Now, I'm not proposing that we can live forever. I am, however, saying that 90% of our medical expenses spent are during the last 10% of our lives. People are no longer dying of simple, natural causes. The majority of deaths globally are related to degenerative processes, and to put it rather bleakly, due to the slow, painful process of neglect. When one can minimize that process, one can live a longer, higher quality of life, especially into older age.

Therefore, the key to overall good health is to determine the relevant factors involved in health correctly. We should always start by managing health at the cellular level. Health is a consequence of choices one has made or has not made. One of my college professors often used to declare, "either you make time for health, or you make time for disease." So, either way, we choose.

A Doctor's Approach to Health

Imagine going to a doctor when you had no issues, no symptoms, nothing. Your blood pressure was acceptable, cholesterol was reasonable, and your weight was appropriate for your age and height. What if, at this visit, you told the doctor that all you wanted to do was maintain this? Hopefully, he or she would say, "great," but they may not be able to offer you much more in the way of maintenance than to say, "keep on doing whatever you're doing." That kind of advice would only work for so long. That is because the medical system is best designed to detect disease early, but not for prevention.

What would you say to an auto mechanic that told you the only maintenance your car required was to have the oil changed at the recommended interval? We know what not getting an oil change on time does to our vehicle. We inherently understand the hassles of repairing the car, insurance claims, or in extreme cases, perhaps even selling it and having to find a new one. Cars are easy, though – as mechanical commodities, we can afford to take them for granted. When we treat our bodies as mechanical commodities, our shelf life shortens dramatically. Indeed a 'use and throw' philosophy, where parts are replaceable and available en masse, does not suit our real-world health.

However, according to the recommendations, if we maintain our bodies in an ideal manner, we can afford to keep them running until we're old and grey. Unfortunately, we don't always give our bodies that TLC. Hopefully, we will have our bodies for many decades, and using this kind of preventative care will prolong their functionality.

Antibiotics & Dis-Ease

Why do we put so little effort into maintaining our bodies? Most people believe that there is a magic pill that will solve all of our problems. Medicine has gone a long way in allowing us to live longer lives; in fact, it has saved millions of lives over time. However, we still age, we still break down, and we still feel pain. In the early stages of dis-ease, the body does the healing; it happens no other way.

The birth of medicine could be attributed to when Robert Koch postulated the germ theory in 1860. Once this discovery took place, it was therefore emphasized and widely believed that microbes were the cause of disease. It was also widely accepted that the key to health was to destroy those foreign enemies. The overuse of antibiotics has created super-strains of bacteria and viruses. These microbes are becoming more resistant to all of the antibiotics designed to fight them off.

Alternative Health Options

People today are becoming increasingly aware of alternatives to medicine. They are sick and tired of being sick and tired, and they want options! They want to know why they are sick or why they are feeling a certain way. They are tired of listening to vague explanations of their issues and question the necessity of taking a pill that will magically solve all their problems. With the abundance of information (some good and some very, very bad) existing on the internet, patients these days are coming in with more confusion than ever.

We *are* getting smarter. For example, in the United States in 2001, there were more visits to Alternative Health Care practitioners than traditional allopathic medical doctors. This statistic was just the tip of the iceberg, as every year since then, this trend has repeated. This may have started with the baby boomers who wanted to create and maintain health, not just mask their problems with drugs and surgery. The flu is not attacking us. We are not innocent victims of evil microbes. With our current lifestyle practices, we are successfully creating a body that is full of toxicity -- the perfect environment for bacteria and viruses to thrive.

Anyone can change their attitude and approach to health. If you continue to look at your body the same way you have in the past, you will continue to get the same results that you always have. However, if you want to change things, you have to start with your mindset. It would be best to prioritize your health. Do not idly take your health for granted; it must be maintained and even improved. If we do something consistently in life, we consider it necessary enough to make it a priority. Therefore, it is essential to look at your health as something so important that it becomes your top priority.

To make your health a priority, you must realize that we make various choices daily that we categorize into two broad areas: doing things that are important and urgent and doing things that are important but not urgent.

Everything in your life that adds meaning or fulfillment is under the category of 'important but not urgent.' Activities such as spending time with your family or significant other, prayer or spirituality, working out, or eating the right foods, all fall under this category.

While these are all very relevant to your overall satisfaction in life, one may not necessarily require them for good health. While eating healthy and exercise are essential elements of health, they aren't usually urgent, of course, depending on the situation.

But what's *urgent* and important? You can think of urgency as a 'house on fire' type of issue. These are time-sensitive things that, if neglected, can do serious harm. An example of this is a yearly physical check-up. If you are over the age of 40 and haven't had a complete physical exam in the last 12 months, I encourage you to make the appointment as soon as possible. No, seriously, put the book down and make the appointment. I'll wait.

Urgency is tied to potential loss if not acted on immediately. Anyone over the age of 18 must commit today. A commitment is part of an urgent/important decision that you'll need to act upon with haste. That commitment is to your overall health in all of your interpersonal capacities. Parent, sibling, colleague, boss, friend, neighbor. You are the only one responsible for your health. Read that again. *YOU are the ONLY ONE responsible for YOUR HEALTH.* Not your wife, not your mom, not your kids. You. Decide to be accountable and committed to your health as an urgent *and* important decision. Luckily, I have some easy tips on how to make this journey less challenging.

The question to ask yourself is, "What can I do today to start on a path of being healthy?" I recommend that my patients start by making changes that are very easy to do. For example, I had a patient who had not exercised in many, many years. I asked her if she could spend 5 minutes a day just stretching. Of course, that sounded very easy to do. Before long, that 5-minute stretch turned into 10 minutes. Next, she realized that the stretching felt good and added some light resistance to her routine with some light weights. At the end of a whole month, she had added cardiovascular exercise to the training and was up to a half-hour of total workout. It was gratifying to see that the habit she created was one she intended on maintaining.

You see, once you create a habit, you can expand upon it, but you will set yourself up for failure if you start too big. Think: short, chunk gains, like biting into a tall sandwich. The most important thing that I want you to get out of this chapter is the subtle consequences our choices have on our health. There are small decisions we make daily that can make the difference between being entirely well or not.

If you would like to test out this theory for yourself, I have an assignment for you. First, we're going to start a 'health journal.' It can be any small notebook that you can keep with you. Next, write down the following on the inside cover or first page of your journal:

"I hereby permit myself to bring my health to the highest level meant to experience, by nurturing myself, by taking care of myself, and by forgiving myself as I would a loved one. I declare today, a day that I will never forget, for it is the day that my life and health changed forever."

Your health journal should begin with a list of goals. Organize these as physical, mental, and spiritual. You may want to eat better, so be specific and list the types of foods you will avoid to obtain better health. If you wish to learn a new skill or improve a relationship, record particular actions you can take and over which you have complete control. The more specific you are, the more successful you will be.

Remember to take your time! This is a deep thought exercise that will tug on your heartstrings. Allow yourself to feel the emotions that may arise, but do not dwell on them. After all, these emotions are arising because they mean something profound to you! Write down as much as you can. It will help you while setting goals later.

Each day, record in your journal or notebook the small steps you have taken. Even record your setbacks and shortcomings because those will help you see your progress over time. There is no such thing as an irreversible mistake now – as long as you document it, you can address the shortcoming and make it right.

How can chiropractic care affect your health?

The most significant way chiropractic can help you is by focusing on the body's ability to regain health, not necessarily dwelling on the symptoms alone. If you constantly chase symptoms, you will never truly recover your body's health potential. You will always be days or months away from your issues reappearing, and you will focus on relieving those symptoms as quickly as possible. It's like putting out fires and never addressing the cause of the blaze. The chances of a new fire starting are high because the cause was never addressed!

As a patient of chiropractic care, you can change your 'standard operating procedure' of going to the doctor only when there is a problem. Instead, you might be going to the chiropractor because you don't want to have any issues in the future or maintain how well you feel. This is a breakthrough in our perceived understanding of health and one that requires time to grasp fully. Consider going to your chiropractor without having pain. Without any symptoms. Without any other purpose other than to *maintain* what is already working correctly. Consider this your regularly scheduled oil change.

Where would we be if we had a health care system in which the doctors were only paid based on how healthy their patients are? The modern medical design has drawn lots of criticism in recent years that echoes its failings in its early years. Alternative medicine was born out of inadequacy of the prevailing system, and similarly, modern medicine earns the moniker of "sick care."

It does not impress me whatsoever when a doctor says, "glad you came in because we just found some major problems in your heart, and we need to go in immediately for a bypass," or something equally extreme. Problems like that never appear out of nowhere. It takes years and years for conditions to develop and get to that severity. Again, we have technology within the medical community that emphasizes early detection at best and very little, if any, prevention. The script is changing slowly, with more doctors prescribing exercise and proper nutrition to combat modern illness. While this is a relatively new strategy in the contemporary medicine playbook, it is the norm with chiropractic care.

You can't just blame the doctors here, either. It is the responsibility of each individual to care for themselves and to take action to prevent disease. Every parent's responsibility is to see that their children are on a path of good, life-long health through preventative care.

How can chiropractic be a strategy to attain health?

The science of chiropractic is in and of itself a fundamental strategy for good health. When you are under chiropractic care, you endeavor to reduce any stress or strain around the spine. This preemptively corrects any issues that could affect the body's ability to adapt to changes internally and externally.

Interference within or surrounding the nervous system causes that dreaded imbalance/dis-ease state or creates a situation where you are not entirely well. Often, you cannot feel that initial interference. There may be no pain or pressure at all to tell you something isn't right. Strangely, the only thing you experience is the imbalance's effects. It may take months or even years for the symptoms to manifest themselves.

It might be easier to understand if you use the example of breast cancer. Did you know that it takes years to create enough density within the breast tissue to see a tumor growth on an X-ray? Sadly, by that time, it may be too late.

Chiropractic does not emphasize waiting for something to go wrong and then arriving heroically to remove the symptom, doing very little about the actual cause of the problem. It focuses on maintaining your natural state of wellness at an optimal level, neurologically speaking.

Think about it this way: if you applied the same rationale to your life in every aspect, would it make your life better, or would it make it worse? If you used the preventative model for your finances, what would it do? If you applied it to your relationship with your spouse, what would that do? All the areas of your life would see a marked improvement. You would no longer be waiting for things to get to the point of being urgent. You would be proactive instead of reactive. You are prioritizing your health as being crucial while not waiting for a crisis to make changes.

The Chiropractic Blueprint to Changing Your Life

The system I am proposing operates on a proper mind-body approach that utilizes two main categories – Information and Empowerment. The changes to make in your life cover different elements of your lifestyle. All this to provide your health with much-needed upkeep. More details to follow in the chapters on nutrition and exercise.

The first aspect of the system involves creative mental processes. Create a mental space and envision a life towards which you would want to aspire. You must have faith in events that you want to have to happen. You should be able to envision these things as both feasible and logical. There should be natural ease about this mental image as if it would lighten your load if it were so.

The second step is to embrace exercise. It is crucially important, and you must take part in it regularly. Stop considering exercise an option, and treat it as a priority. Can't exercise because you've already put in tons of energy at work? Exercise before work. Are you pooped from chasing the kids around the house? Take the chasing outside and cover some ground. All tuckered out from putting in work in the garden? Stretch it out once your job is complete.

Despite looking and feeling like exercise, none of these excuses stand up as a proper workout. You must have cardiovascular training for health – movement that tests and drives your heart harder. Your heart comprises of cardiac muscle, and its sole purpose is to pump blood through your entire body every day, all day, no days off. Keeping it as strong as possible is the healthiest option for such a vital organ.

The third element of this blueprint is to learn how breathing correctly is of utmost importance. Breathing provides oxygen to the tissues of the body. Oxygen works down from the organ level (lungs) to the tissues and eventually nourishes every cell within the body. The lungs are just the port. As mentioned earlier, the lack of oxygen to the cells is one reason for cell dysfunction. Breathe for balance, ease, and good health!

The fourth important factor is hydration. Staying hydrated is necessary to flush out toxins from the body and keep the shape of your cells. Your body is composed of 75% water, not 75% coffee, tea, or soda! Despite giving you an illusion of energy, these popular water replacements do not have many health benefits (even though caffeine addicts like me may object to this statement!) The academic community is split on this idea of thirst. Some say that once you feel thirsty, you may be up to 10% dehydrated already. Others say that the body does a reasonably good job of staying hydrated, so no minimum should be observed. Again, the theory of preventative maintenance works here. A minimum of 2L of water a day is optimal for *basic* health purposes. For *good* health, aim for about 3L every day. At first, you may need to pee quite often but think of it as beneficial detoxification each time you flush.

The following fundamental truth is about greens. As children, many avoided micronutrient-packed roughage at all costs, not understanding the magnitude of their nutritional value. Eating plenty of green, leafy vegetables every week is one of the most effective things you can do for yourself. Plants create energy to survive through photosynthesis, a complex set of reactions that converts sunlight to a usable form of nutrition. The potency of the nutrients in fresh leafy greens is among the highest in the world of food. Most importantly, consume more raw vegetables, or you stand to lose out on tons of nutrients. Overcooking of raw plants destroys the necessary enzymes to break down plant material. These enzymes are vital to good health.

One more thing you should add to your diet is a healthy amount of antioxidants. These biochemicals allow you to minimize the ravaging effects of free radicals within us, increasing in number as we age. Consuming processed foods can start the production of free radicals. They spawn in times of stress and during injury. Without intervention, free radicals can create havoc at the cell's level. Increased infections, lowered immunity, dis-ease, and disease can all result due to these damaged cells.

Fats and oils are perhaps the least understood macronutrients. Fats (made up of fatty acids) are required so that your body has sufficient oil levels to make the membrane surrounding each cell.

This outer layer comprises a double layer called a bi-phospholipid layer, which allows essential molecules and materials into the cell while keeping unwanted items out.

The main issue with fats and oils in the diet is that many people consume too much of the wrong type of fats. 90% of people, according to researchers, are deficient in consuming these 'correct' oils. This fact is interesting since cardiovascular disease and the resulting list of degenerative disorders were always thought to occur due to overly fatty diets. The truth is, not all fats are created equal. All foods that contain fat include a variety of them. The following is a short breakdown of the types of oils that are available in our food:

Unsaturated fats (monounsaturated and polyunsaturated)

Omega-3

Saturated fats

Trans fats

Avoid saturated and trans fats to the greatest extent possible. Unsaturated fats are liquid at room temperature, and we should consume them actively. This is especially true for Omega-3s. Since the body does not manufacture them, we must ingest them. So, believe it or not, good oils are by far the best heart disease-preventative measure that you can take.

The last proactive step that you need to take is to maintain a healthy nervous system. Think about this for a moment. If you were consuming everything that I recommended, and yet your nervous system was not functioning correctly, would the signal from the brain allot nutrient resources appropriately? How well would the signaling to the cell carry out internal processes?

According to researchers, the standard impulse transmission for nerves can reduce by up to 60%, with pressure from a weight of only two grams! This tiny amount of pressure significantly impacts the body's ability to send and receive messages by so much. If you continue to evaluate the choices you make regularly, install the ideas we've talked about, and maintain your body, your outlook will look exceptionally healthy! Cultivating a positive mental attitude and focusing your beliefs on prevention rather than fixing problems once they occur is a more challenging step but can be accomplished with practice. Eating well with various fresh, raw vegetables and fruits, good fats, and tons of antioxidants is a great starting point for any "get healthy" goals. Staying hydrated and exercising are the uncomplicated changes you can make right now. Visiting your chiropractor to take care of your nervous system and keep you on track with your health goals is probably the easiest step of all!

Chapter 4

Blending Chiropractic Care with Traditional Medicine

A survey of people seeking alternative care shows that of all methods, they choose chiropractic most often. Most chiropractors recognize the value of combined or multidisciplinary healthcare treatments. Unfortunately, the same sentiment does not reciprocate in the medical profession as a whole. While a portion of chiropractors feel that this discipline can and should treat all types of illnesses and injuries, most recognize the role of traditional and modern medical practices. Inroads have been made in bridging the gap between mainstream medicine and so-called 'alternative' methods. However, bringing patients the best of overall health requires some further work.

The philosophy of multidisciplinary healthcare is a step-by-step approach, starting with the least invasive and, if necessary, gradually working toward more invasive and aggressive treatments. An example may be in the case of a patient with vague low back pain. Suppose there is no relief after receiving a complete chiropractic assessment and some treatment for possible pressure on nerves related to the area. In that case, the chiropractor refers to the appropriate medical professional for imaging. If this same patient were to begin their care with an Orthopedic Doctor, they might have walked out of that office with a prescription in hand to treat back pain symptoms, never really exploring the *cause* of the symptoms.

There are genuine and thorough doctors who don't automatically prescribe medication but further explore the reasons behind the symptoms. Unfortunately, they can be challenging to find. Especially in a country like India, where most hospitals are run for-profit, it becomes exceedingly hard to find quality care from physicians who want to improve patients' health more than meeting minimum billing quotas.

The final and least desirable of any treatment is, of course, surgery. Back surgery may ultimately be a prescription for a damaged disc, but perhaps all that patient needed was a spinal adjustment. If the nerve signals were unblocked and communicated clearly to the back's pain-producing area, the patient could have avoided surgery. Chiropractic treatment and a care plan on how to take care of this injury into the future could prevent the need for surgery in this patient forever. I've seen hundreds of these same cases already. While it may seem impressive to some, chiropractors worldwide would not bat an eyelash at these results. To us, these 'miracles' are literally just another day at the office.

The number of medical doctors that refer their patients to chiropractors is still disappointingly low. However, we're increasingly seeing chiropractors getting invites to attend and speak at medical conferences and write for medical journals. These are two forums medical doctors use to keep current with breakthroughs in medicine and treatment methods. Chiropractors are putting a more concerted effort into scientific research and are holding higher ranking positions in the medical world. It is, perhaps, the role of patients and chiropractors alike to keep educating medical doctors on the benefits of the less invasive methods of chiropractic. The message is of unity and of providing the best options available for healthcare to the patient.

Massage & Chiropractic

Many doctors send patients for massage therapy following an injury, neck, or back pain. Massage can be amazingly effective in relieving the pain, especially if the cause is muscular.

Many chiropractors have come to incorporate massage therapy into their practices. There has been evidence that regular massages help maintain the positive results of chiropractic adjustments. The stimulation of the muscles improves muscle tone and function, especially along the spinal column.

Tense muscles also negatively impact the spinal column by pulling on the vertebrae. This tension, especially on muscles attached to the spine, can restrict the spinal joint and diminish the function of the nearby nerves.

There are several other benefits of deep tissue and other types of massage. If you have ever had a good massage, the therapist should have instructed you to drink plenty of water following the session. The reason for this is massage facilitates lymphatic circulation and allows the body to release various toxins. It is, therefore, vital to flush out those toxins with lots of clean water.

Massage can also help increase peripheral circulation and vascular circulation in the arms and legs. Because these systems supply the heart with oxygen-rich blood, improving circulation is always beneficial. These functions, along with the drainage of the lymphatic system, rid the body of waste and strengthen the immune system.

Finally, and perhaps most commonly, massage can reduce stress. Any emotional or physical stress hurts the full function of the body. Human beings are generally receptive to touch, and studies have shown the benefit of therapeutic touch, as in massage. A well-trained massage therapist can be an integral member of your overall health and wellness team.

Physiotherapy & Chiropractic

Many parallels exist between physiotherapy and Chiropractic, and the gap between the two professions continues to shorten. *Physiotherapy* or *physical therapy* is the profession of physical rehabilitation experts and occupies a role in the healthcare world similar to chiropractors.

Physiotherapists help patients who are usually suffering from pain of some origin, mechanically, neurologically, developmentally, or otherwise. They are generally deployed on injuries of various forms and work with patients from all walks of life. They are an integral member of all healthcare systems and can make the difference from hospital to home.

I have always had a strong inclination to work alongside physiotherapists and currently include them in our multidisciplinary approach to healthcare. They are talented rehabilitation experts and can provide the necessary critical evaluation and instruction needed for patients to develop the motor control required to overcome their injuries.

The difference between chiropractors and physiotherapists stems from the training provided. In North America, there is an even more significant overlap between the two professions, with physiotherapists earning a Doctorate of Physical Therapy (DPT). The skillset demonstrated by well-trained physiotherapists can rival even the most accomplished chiropractors.

The main difference between Chiropractic and physiotherapy is the manual technique employed, namely the chiropractic adjustment, a systematic method to assess and align the spine using manual manipulation. Chiropractors have long-held beliefs that the chiropractic adjustment is the one element that keeps our profession separate and distinct from other healthcare disciplines. Courses and certifications have been popping up worldwide, further decreasing the skill gap between chiropractors and physiotherapists. Again, to emphasize this point, chiropractors receive far more expertise in manipulating the spine through their doctoral education.

Chiropractors around the world are also adapting to changing healthcare environments. Entire thought processes and learning streams have evolved to include deeply scientific and detail-oriented movement assessments and screenings. More chiropractors involve thorough rehabilitation instructions and exercises for their patients to augment the care they provide through adjustments and alignments.

Another considerable difference between chiropractors and physiotherapists is the ability of Chiropractors to examine, assess, diagnose and treat any patient that walks into their office. Chiropractors are primary care doctors who do not require any previous referral from another primary care practitioner. New changes notwithstanding, physiotherapists (in North America) can only treat patients referred to them.

A Chiropractic Wellness Program

Chiropractic should be incorporated into everybody's health care. If you have a spine, you need a chiropractor. As one of the least invasive forms of healthcare, it derives from the principles that the body can heal independently, with lessened interference in communication between brain and body. Once again, the idea of wellness crops up and relates to the concept of preventative care. Once we have attained better health, we should aim to preserve it, and with it, sustain a better and happier life.

The average healthy person does not place enough emphasis on preventative care. Think about it: If you were to have fewer aches and pains, less of a problem with waking up in the morning, more energy because you feel 100%, wouldn't the quality of your life be better? A routine of regular chiropractic care can provide this.

Chiropractic checkups can provide a boost for most generally healthy people. It isn't about back pain or orthopedic injuries.

Essentially, it's about keeping the lines of communication open for messages the nerves send to the rest of the body. This way, chiropractic care can correct what isn't entirely right or prevent any issues potentially around the corner. As we age, degeneration is inevitable but becomes slower with routine adjustments.

The Cost of Chiropractic Care

Many people who are not wholly aware of the benefits of chiropractic may be reluctant to start a wellness program simply because of the cost. These costs vary across the globe. A typical chiropractic visit is slightly higher in price than a visit to a general practitioner in India, but that dynamic is the opposite in the western world. While healthcare costs in India continue to skyrocket, value is a word that often gets tossed around. As alluded to previously, the country runs with a for-profit model in the hospital industry, which means everything you do gets billed. In many cases, the doctors receive incentives for higher billing.

Health insurance is also a relatively new addition to the healthcare landscape in India, with many companies now offering very affordable premiums. Unfortunately, chiropractic care has yet to become widely available within these plans and may take a few more years for empanelment. In western countries, health insurance is one of the primary ways patients opt to pay for their chiropractic care. Since many multinational companies with headquarters in India originated from the US, speak to your insurance provider about whether chiropractic care is covered.

If your insurance company does not cover chiropractic care, don't panic; you will be pleased to know that it *is* affordable, especially when you look at the alternative. With a focus on prevention and a look at lifestyle, many chiropractors also offer family plans, care plans, or session 'packages' at reduced rates. We all want you to continue your health care in this positive, preventative manner, so we make it as easy as possible.

The Doctor-Patient Relationship

Any health examination is a highly personal interaction. I'm sure you can envision the situation: two people who meet, perhaps for the first time, sit together in a room. One tells the other what kinds of activities they are involved in to break the ice, then starts talking about their body – where it hurts, what past illnesses they have had, and any problems they have with normal functions of the body. Pretty personal stuff. Next, the other person says something like, "Well, lie down, let me take a look."

Chiropractic care is similar to any other kind of medical care, only because there is complete confidentiality between doctor and patient. The similarities, however, end there. When you create a relationship with a Doctor of Chiropractic, it will be personal, but in a manner you may not have thought of before. Chiropractic care is specific to the individual in that it takes a look at the whole person. Chiropractors examine not only the identifiable aches and pains or illnesses but the entire lifestyle, family situation, occupation, and concerns even outside the realm of your health.

A very few such physicians take the time and care enough to learn about every aspect of the patient's life. With chiropractors, however, it is more a norm than an exception. Studies show that the level of satisfaction with chiropractors far surpassed all other health care practitioners. This fact was observable over patient outcomes, reasons for visit, and value for a visit. Some medical doctors see patients for less than 1 minute!

Upon regular or even infrequent visits to the chiropractor, you will find that a basis of trust becomes established, and a very high level of concern applies to each visit. These facts alone may be the reason why chiropractic care seems to be a family affair. Many patients will return with their spouses, children, and best friends because they are completely comfortable and satisfied with the personal attention during chiropractic treatment.

When was the last time you went to a medical doctor and received personal attention? It's not very common. Chiropractic care works on the ability to reach each person and treat them as an individual. The treatments may 'look' the same for everybody, but there is a large degree of nuance dedicated to each patient's specific needs. Your results are our results, and we take a certain amount of pride in restoring you to the optimal version of yourself. This is why your Chiropractor will usually remember your interests, hobbies, or even ask how your last round of golf went without looking it up! We care about you!

You're Visit to the Chiropractor

If you are new to the wonder of chiropractic, you may be a little unsure about what to expect. Is there going to be some massage-like table slab where I lay down to have someone pound my back and crack my spine? Do I have to get undressed? Is there anyone else in the room with me during an examination or adjustment? These are all perfect questions, which, if left unanswered, could dissuade someone from visiting a chiropractor.

You may be surprised to know that a visit to the chiropractor is one of the most relaxing and comfortable types of health care visits – and I can almost guarantee it hurts less than going to the dentist: physically, emotionally, and financially.

When you enter the chiropractor's office, you will be greeted by a warm receptionist ready to answer your questions and get some information from you. You will complete some paperwork on your health history, your current complaints, and register on our highly confidential record-keeping system.

Depending on your issues and symptoms, the healing can begin even on your first visit, as a light and gentle adjustment or manipulation to your spinal column may occur. That's not the focus initially, though. This is a time for gathering information, including a comprehensive medical history, and for the chiropractor to listen to what concerns you. It is a time to establish trust, make you comfortable, and discuss what possible therapy could benefit you.

Our trained professionals will take you through a series of tests and assessments and then present a plan of action depending on the issues discussed. Sometimes, it's required to get some medical tests or imaging done before the treatment can occur. Although this may be part of the billing racket of other practices, this is only to come to the most concise and practical treatment plan for you. We want you to be safe and happy throughout your treatment, so sometimes, understanding a bit more about the body requires further testing.

Chiropractors often face the same issues regularly, so it is common practice to make similar recommendations for similar conditions. As mentioned before, we take pride in personalizing treatment for each patient and ensuring safety above all else.

Here is some general advice for your first visit for those considering making an appointment with your local chiropractor. In general, it is wise to have your medical documents (if any) up to date, in order, and accessible. Bring them to your appointment as they can give your chiropractor valuable insight into your issues, even if you don't feel like they are relevant. Definitely bring all medical imaging and testing, and leave it to the chiropractor to decide if it requires consideration.

Secondly, it is advisable to have a warm shower before attending your session. Definitely helpful in terms of hygiene and courtesy; it can also help your muscles relax, which will be beneficial if any treatment happens. Wearing loose, stretchy, or generally comfortable clothes is also advisable. If the clothing is restrictive to the necessary procedures, a change of clothes may be available at the clinic. Alternatively, bringing a pair of shorts and a t-shirt to your appointment may also be convenient.

Being early to your first appointment is advisable, as you may have lots of information to input, and the registration could take slightly longer as a result. Planning to have extra time to locate the clinic, find parking, and relax before the appointment is beneficial. Being in a rush can add stress to an already new experience, to which you may already have some fears. Take it easy! We're here to help.

Following the recommendations is always advisable. Understanding the doctor's instructions is essential, so make sure you have asked the questions you wanted to ask before the end of your appointment. Many people jot down their questions in a notebook or on their phones as reminders. Calling the clinic to speak with the doctor may not always be possible in the midst of a full schedule of patients, so being prepared goes a long way to getting the answers you desire.

In my practice, our policy is to ensure end-to-end care from the moment you enter our office to the moment you leave. Each practitioner methodically goes through their recommendations and explains each step of the process. In many cases, follow-up care is suggested to track progress and quickly address new developments.

A lengthier care plan may be recommended in some instances, as some issues require more time to heal. If this is the case, make sure you understand the treatment goals and what the doctor needs from your end. Most commonly, pain is why patients come to the clinic and are amazed to see that their pain disappears in just a couple of sessions. Despite promising early results, their treatment plan continues. Remember this – pain is just the tip of the iceberg – it is most often the *last* thing to show up and the *first* thing to disappear. The *cause* of the pain is really what your chiropractor is trying to fix, which might take more time. Stick with the plan. It works!

Chapter 5

Chiropractic Credentials – Are Chiropractors Doctors?

If you have ever had any doubts about whether or not chiropractors are qualified to provide the crucial type of healthcare services rendered by this profession, this chapter should set your mind at ease. Doctors of Chiropractic (DC, the official title given once education and clinical training are complete) receive just about as much classroom education in biology, physiology, and other sciences as medical doctors. One significant difference between MD (Medical Doctor) programs and DC programs is the concentration of subject material. MD programs are heavier in pharmacology and toxicology (think: medicine), while DC programs load up on anatomy and radiology (think: the physical body). Because the DC program is non-allopathic and involves manual techniques, a good proportion of the program includes kinesthetic laboratory training. Both MD and DC programs have a similar amount of coursework in patient assessment and clinical diagnosis.

A student attending an accredited chiropractic college starts with an average of four years of college-level course work in a pre-medical, scientific field. Upon entering the chiropractic college curriculum, the student begins the journey of another minimum of

4,200 hours of classroom, laboratory, and clinical training. The majority of this time gets spent in a clinical setting.

It is challenging to learn to adjust the spine and master the necessary pressure and delicate balance of touch without hands-on experience. Once the classroom training has allowed the student to become knowledgeable on the functions and form of the body, the clinical experience prepares them to make accurate and precise adjustments. While each college is slightly different in delivering this training, my alma mater - New York Chiropractic College -included hands-on coursework from the moment we started the program. The early coursework allowed us to understand landmarks on the body and the idea of using our body to move another person. It also made us very disciplined in our bedside manner – the empathetic professionalism maintained while speaking to patients about their issues.

This kind of schooling also ranks Doctors of Chiropractic among the highest trained health care professionals. Here is a good comparison of the hours spent in training by a chiropractor and a medical student. There are many different numbers out there that vary from one medical school or chiropractic college to the next, so this chart summarizes the averages of several sources.

Subjects	Class Hours Chiropractic Students	Class Hours Medical Students
Anatomy	540	510
Chemistry	165	325
Diagnosis	630	325
Microbiology	120	115
Neurology	320	110
Obstetrics	60	150
Orthopedics	210	155
Pathology	360	400
Physiology	240	325
Psychiatry	60	145
Radiology	360	150
HOURS	3,065	2,710

ADDITIONALLY REQUIRED STUDIES

Chiropractic School	Medical School
Spinal Manipulation Nutrition Physiotherapy Advanced Radiology	Pharmacology Immunology General Surgery

Colleges of chiropractic that are accredited have obtained the approval of the Council on Chiropractic Education. United States Department of Education recognizes this council, as do many other international education authorities. There are currently 46 accredited colleges of chiropractic or programs within academic institutions around the world today. Programs outside the United States are certified by local governing boards of the educational accreditation organizations for those countries.

Board Exams and Agencies Governing Chiropractic Care.

One of the best ways for any group of people to be held accountable to uphold a high standard of performance is to let their peers monitor them. Chiropractic has had a hard enough time gaining acceptance among some mainstream healthcare professionals, so it would be even more difficult if it were not for its strict requirements on licensing imposed by other chiropractors and the government.

The process of watching over the chiropractic profession begins with education and training. Schools of chiropractic can only become accredited by an agency entirely accepted and recognized by the local branch of education regulations (ex. U.S. Department of Education). Students from this system graduate well-trained and prepared to practice chiropractic, but it doesn't stop there. Licensing in all 50 states in the United States and by agencies worldwide occurs to make sure Doctors of Chiropractic are capable of doing whatever their scope of practice outlines. Any field impacting a person's health and well-being should be licensed and certified. Chiropractic is no exception.

National and state examinations are necessary to determine if a chiropractor is qualified to treat patients. This is a four-part test in the US, a three-part test in Canada, and other jurisdictions enforce their specific regulations. Doctors of Chiropractic in most locales must participate in a certain number of continuing education hours each year to keep their license current. This policy also ensures that your chiropractor is up to date on new advances in the profession, new codes of conduct that become enforceable, and knowledgeable of the legislations governing chiropractic practice.

State licensing agencies are operational at state divisions of occupational licensing and boards of chiropractic examiners located regionally. They are the watchdogs for the field so that only the top, most qualified chiropractors can work with patients. They are also in charge of hearing complaints, arbitration on professional grievances, and other housekeeping measures within the profession. The members of these councils are typically elected, adding further dimensions of fairness and policy.

Chiropractors are also part of a community of other chiropractors and can learn and further develop their skills through professional trade associations specific to chiropractic. Some of these organizations have programs recognized by the Council on Chiropractic Education that provide detailed, specialized training in particular subcategories of chiropractic. Doctors of Chiropractic can become certified as specialists in orthopedics, neurology, occupational and industrial health, diagnostic testing, internal disorders, imaging thermography, and sports injury. These specialties may help a patient decide on a potential chiropractor, specifically if their specialization is in an area of concern for the patient.

I graduated from New York Chiropractic College in 2012, where I was an active student leader. On top of the rigorous program of study, I made the most of my time by becoming a Teaching Assistant, working with the Admissions office and the Alumni office, and volunteering with research projects run at the College. I also found time to run the first edition of the Canadian Chiropractic Club, which still functions today! All these activities and generally good grades helped me win Student of the Year. I won a few more awards at graduation, but I was happier to know that my experience at NYCC shaped me to be a great clinician.

The clinical part of the program was fantastic. I felt that I was raising the bar on how impactfully I could help my patient at every turn. As I had mentioned earlier, from the word go, the clinical curriculum was front and center. We were constantly aware of how our bodies played a role in our ability to perform chiropractic adjustments. The various classes drove home all the cues towards a professional bedside manner. What truly moved the needle for my experience was the vast array of course options we had to explore. We could become any kind of clinician we wanted; the choice was ours.

My inclination was towards soft tissue work. Under other clinicians and my own experiences with being adjusted, I had come to realize that you could not ignore the soft tissue element. I loaded up my electives with technique courses that offered guidance and theory to various soft-tissue methods. I was so well-versed in these courses that I assisted a professor in teaching a soft-tissue technique.

The clinical rotations were also challenging and helped increase my confidence, moving from backpack to briefcase, so to speak. As a student intern, I would never have imagined having the courage to work on some of the fascinating cases that came through. However, with the support and guidance of expert clinical supervisors, we witnessed firsthand what our abilities could help achieve.

One of my favorite memories and experiences was from a clinical rotation at a Veterans Administration in Canandaigua, New York. I was assigned a patient whose military career consisted of over 250 jumps from over 10,000 feet. The retired paratrooper's spine was a mess, littered with old compression fractures and disc herniations. After working on him for a couple of weeks, curiosity got the better of me, and I asked, "am I even helping you? I mean, you come in every day with the same type of thing." He looked at me, then very slowly, he smiled. He said, "If you've been wondering why I've been coming down almost every day, it's because you have been the first person who's made me feel good enough to not take 2 of my pain killers." A quick look at his prescription history told me he was on a painkiller cocktail from which even Jordan Belfort would avoid. It struck me at that moment; I couldn't cure this guy. But that didn't mean that I couldn't help him.

Chapter 6

Diagnostic Methods Used in Chiropractic

Chiropractic is like other medical practices, where although the process is similar, small things will differ from clinic to clinic. A typical patient evaluation and history taking are in line with traditional medicine, as this discovers the most pertinent information around a condition. Chiropractors train to take histories and use diagnostic tools to narrow down and differentiate between problems that can manifest similar symptoms.

Some of the standard tests used in chiropractic are orthopedic and neurological. These measures usually include X-rays, ultrasound, range of motion, and mobility analysis. In some cases where a patient presents with nerve-related issues, blood vessel or circulatory issues, or clues to visceral pathology, MRIs, CT scans, and doppler images are necessary. Every jurisdiction has its own rules about what medical imaging a chiropractor can and cannot order for, so in certain situations, a chiropractor may need to refer to a medical doctor for a patient to get the tests they need.

There is also a hands-on analysis where a trained chiropractor can feel obvious misalignments in the spine and other joints. They can tell through touch when vertebrae have shifted to the point where there may be interference with the neurological signals transmitted by the spinal nerves. This practice is called *palpation* or *motion palpation.* The movement of each joint has a normal range, and chiropractors can assess these joints to evaluate for any restricted motion.

There are also some cutting-edge technological advancements brought to light by the growing field of chiropractic. Working with established instrumentation and combining it with the newest technology allows chiropractors to picture the entire situation before recommending and beginning any treatment. Certain advances have improved patient outcomes, while others have increased the ability of the patient to understand how they have benefited from chiropractic care.

'Subluxation Stations'

This kind of instrument used in chiropractic can offer a complete look and analyze where and what type of issue occurs in the patient. It uses a static surface electromyogram (sEMG) to measure electrical activity. This activity is then run through software to create a color map where the pressure on a nerve is taking place.

The colorful illustration displayed as output results from any electrical activity in the muscles around the spine. It measures paraspinal infrared temperature to assess the spine's range of motion automatically. The unit also measures pain around the spine. This system is one of the most effective methods of communicating the spine's issues, especially the asymptomatic stress that may be present.

Thermal Imaging Instruments

Chiropractors use infrared imaging to view changes in temperature where soft-tissue injuries may have occurred. It can also measure increases in pain and then treat these areas with infrared light therapy, which increases blood circulation to the region. It can even stimulate cellular and nerve function painlessly.

A process called Computerized Infrared Thermography (CIT) uses a handheld paraspinal scanner. The device scans and generates graphs that are laid one over the other for analysis and comparison.

The Nervo-Scope

This instrument is used both before and after the chiropractor makes any adjustments to the patient's spine. Before the manipulation, the scope assesses temperature readings taken along the spine. Following the adjustment, the readings are again recorded to measure the difference. This method allows the chiropractor to see how much of a reduction in spinal restriction has occurred. Famous chiropractor and industry trail-blazer Dr. Clarence Gonstead brought the use of this technique to the forefront. Today, you can see the nervo-scope in action on YouTube in videos from famous personalities like "Dr. Rahim."

The Myogauge

This trademarked instrument primarily measures the range of motion and isometric muscle strength for any body part. The systems are highly customized, so each practitioner can add the accessories that best serve their patients. The computerized system documents the results from digitally measuring the amount of force created by the patient's movements.

Regional Spinal Testing

There are instruments used in chiropractic that focus on the various regions of the spinal column, measuring and recording such results as temperature and the waveform created by the spine. One such instrument is the Pro-Adjuster which taps each segment of the spine to gather its objective data.

Other instruments used in spinal screening incorporate bilateral weight and postural evaluations. Taking a deep dive into the complex technology associated with chiropractic diagnosis highlights the advances that have transpired over the years. A visit to the chiropractor is not just a bone-cracking session based on hit or miss adjustments. This passage also illustrates that many practices have different systems aimed at the same thing – excellent patient outcomes! For patients who have experienced incredible results with a chiropractor using one method, going to another clinic using a different system might feel "wrong." For these situations, realize that each technology used is for improving some element of the process and may have no effect on the *quality* of your care.

The spine is one of, if not THE most important, system in the body. No legitimate, well-trained chiropractor is going to proceed with manipulations blindly. Highly sophisticated instrumentation and diagnostic tools are available to make educated, necessary adjustments and help document objective progress.

In my practice, we use several different tools to help the patient understand their body better. While the availability of some of these technologies in India is nil, we have still done our best to acquire more commercially available equipment. All our clinics have the latest electronic posture analysis software and biometric scanners for your vital statistics. Clinically we are well prepared to provide over ten different chiropractic techniques. These techniques help diagnose a wide range of misalignments that can be preventing complete wellness. They can see a potential problem long before the patient ever experiences any symptoms.

Chapter 7

What Should You Look for In a Chiropractor?

There is no question that who you choose as a chiropractor is just as (if not more) personal as selecting a medical doctor. It is the same type of scrutiny you would use when looking for someone to be an integral part of your overall wellness plan. Provided you have a goal that will enable you to live your life to the fullest; a chiropractor would be an excellent fit.

Since Doctors of Chiropractic are required to complete more than 4,200 hours of classroom, laboratory, and clinical training, they come from that training well prepared and qualified to care for you and your family. So the deciding factor for you may be more based on such subjective criteria as location, personality traits, gender, and practice policies. Most people today in India recognize the importance of preventative healthcare, and some are finding out about the role of chiropractic. In India, the number of certified Chiropractors is few, and on average, their prices are lower than the world average. In the US, most employees of companies are covered for some degree of their healthcare by insurance. Some of these multinational companies (MNC) extend these benefits to their Indian employees, so cost is less of a concern in choosing a chiropractor.

More than 100,000 Doctors of Chiropractic practice across 90 countries worldwide, and the numbers are quickly growing. Finding one close to home is limited to a few choices at the moment, but more options should be available soon. The problem then becomes deciding which of your neighborhood chiropractic offices meets your needs.

Types of Chiropractors

Not all chiropractors are the same. There are, in fact, two general types of chiropractors with slightly differing views on how chiropractic fits into a plan for health and wellness. There are some philosophical differences between these two camps, but both styles of chiropractic function entirely for the patient's benefit. There is a spectrum of options between these two extremes, and most modern chiropractors understand the basics of both styles.

Some view chiropractic as the only form of healthcare necessary for good health and treating all ailments. This group performs procedures to specifically remove "subluxations" in the body to free the nerve signal passed down from the brain to the body and vice versa. Subluxation in this context refers to an obstruction or blockage, usually from the vertebral column, and not the traditional medical term for 'dislocation.' The 'adjustment' of the subluxation, in turn, allows the body to heal itself by sending the correct information to the corresponding parts of the body. This type of chiropractor is referred to as a "straight chiropractor."

The second type of chiropractor is called a "mixer." In their practices, they combine traditional straight chiropractic with other forms of natural healthcare. For example, mixers may employ physical modalities such as electrical stimulations, massage, or hot-and-cold therapies to relieve pain and stimulate the body to heal and recuperate. A big part of a mixer's view on health is nutrition and exercise and their roles in maintaining a healthy spine and nervous system.

In my practice, I don't necessarily categorize myself as one or the other. Still, I have had colleagues refer to my practice as definitely 'mixer.' The background to this turf war within the profession tends to get ugly, as one group's beliefs are mutually exclusive of the other's. I see value in both styles and philosophies.

I use modalities and soft tissue methods in my practice, which is frowned upon by the so-called "Principled" or straight chiropractors. I rely on exercise and rehabilitation to ensure my patients are empowered and not dependent on getting adjusted multiple times every week. Again, not something the Straights would approve.

The mixer group is getting more vocal in their intolerance for the Straights. The Mixers portray the "scientific arm" of chiropractic, adhering so steadfastly to the results of research that many people aren't considered patients of this style. Robotically sticking to a method has its limitations as well. Since evidence-based chiropractic (EBC) is exceedingly difficult to produce en masse, the holes in the overall strategy are numerous.

This issue is very "yin yang" in my mind. The mixers feel like the straights are anachronistically holding on to theories of the past. The straights believe the mixers will lose the essence of what makes chiropractic different from all other health practices. Jargon like 'subluxation,' 'adjustment,' 'innate intelligence,' and others are sneered at by the mixers. Any practice outside spinal manipulation is blasphemy to the chiropractic dogma - warn the straights. And on and on it goes.

Once, I had a gang of straight chiropractic students confront me about my beliefs. My college, NYCC, is notorious among straight colleges for being "extra mixer" – and I was on campus at a straight college in California for a conference. I had a target on my back as soon as I landed. So, during one of the student outings, I was asked if I was a mixer. I deferred answering. They persisted. They taunted me about not knowing the philosophy and never reading "The Green Books" (a manifesto written by one of Chiropractic's founders and key influencer, BJ Palmer). I never saw the benefit of labeling myself. Either way, one group was not going to be happy. So, amidst the growing commotion surrounding my official stance, I silenced the crowd with a simple statement – "I do what I do as a Chiropractor to help my patient in whatever way I can. If that's not what we're supposed to do, call me whatever you like."

Other Characteristics in a Chiropractor

Some may be looking for a female Doctor of Chiropractic instead of a male. You may want someone who is especially good with children if you plan to start your child's healthcare regime with regular chiropractic care. There are also personality traits to consider since some people just get along and feel more comfortable with certain people. Even though the choice of which chiropractor to visit is a personal one, there is security in knowing that the governing bodies are constantly doing their jobs to make sure your practitioner is fully licensed and qualified to provide chiropractic care.

One trait you will very often find in a chiropractor is their focus on family. Unlike myself, many chiropractors are second or third-generation Doctors of Chiropractic. Most have been to a chiropractor from a young age. It could very well be that chiropractic is a typical family business. In some cases, children of chiropractors become Doctors of Chiropractic themselves because they have been taught and realize the importance of chiropractic to overall health and well-being. A child of a chiropractor will often tell new patients that their first adjustment was just moments after birth to correct any misalignments that may have occurred during the birthing process. This gentle handling of an infant's spine will ensure all systems are optimal for the new life ahead.

In my practice, one of the first patients in Bangalore I was lucky to work with was a lady who was five months pregnant. She had a great experience throughout her life with chiropractic and continued her care with me. I adjusted her well into her pregnancy and adjusted her the night before she went into labor. On visiting the family in the hospital, she handed me the infant and asked if I wanted to adjust him! A quick check of the spine revealed a happy, healthy baby boy and resulted in a joy I've never quite felt before. It is an absolute, singular, and unimaginable delight to have earned that trust with someone. Imagine someone who went through all kinds of stress and pain for nine months, pushed through it, and then hands you this beautiful baby to check for any issues. I'll never forget that moment for the rest of my life. To say that our profession is rewarding is an understatement of epic proportions!

There are different types of chiropractors, just like there are different types of medical doctors. In the medical field, some doctors specialize in pediatrics, neurology, or endocrinology. The same is true for chiropractors, but with some subtle differences. Picking a chiropractor that possesses additional skills or training in your specific issue can be a determining factor.

All chiropractors receive the same general chiropractic education and training for the specialty of chiropractic – no matter what other course of study they may have pursued before the specialized chiropractic college curriculum. The college program is similar to a general medical practitioner gaining an education in all body systems, then specializing in something more specific. General knowledge of all the correct functions of the body is studied so that when something is wrong, they know just which specialist gets their referral.

Throughout the history of the world, there have been "alternative" methods of healthcare. Ancient Chinese medicine, considered the only treatment at the time, is making a comeback in some healthcare regimens. For some chiropractic practitioners, the chiropractic form of health care is used instead of any other type of intervention. It is considered complete on its own. Some believe that the root cause of all disease is through the first bone in the spine, the

Atlas. This belief is probably the most extreme and narrowly focused philosophy of "straight" practitioners.

A 1998 study (reference found at the end of the book) of how the average person utilized chiropractic care indicated that the reasons for going to a chiropractor were varied. The study by Hurwitz looked at the records of 5,000 chiropractic offices and found more than 130 different diagnoses. Most (13.7%) still dealt with sprains and strains of the spine and other musculoskeletal systems. A small percentage of patients recognized chiropractic could do so much more. A total of 3.6% went for reasons such as headache, migraines, asthma, and myalgia.

On the other end of the spectrum is the Chiropractor that deals strictly with neck pain, back pain, and injuries. These may be patients with chronic pain (pain lasting longer than six months) or those who have been in a recent car accident. Another common injury category is the "weekend warrior" who just lifted a piece of furniture the wrong way during an all-day cleaning binge or played 4 hours of pickup basketball in their driveway with no warm-up or cool down. Their practice and procedures may be purely therapeutic and involve a finite number of treatments until the pain is better managed or eliminated.

While most of my practice is the latter, someone experiencing pain for any reason, I extend to see patients with slightly broader issues. Our office utilizes an integrated healthcare model, where multiple eyes and clinical opinions are better than one person dictating for all. Often, patients who attend for musculoskeletal issues ask questions about other problems someone they know might have.

We usually encourage all such patients to visit for a consultation. After a more thorough understanding of the issue, we offer our expertise, whether through treatment or referral to another practitioner.

Back pain, neck pain, and headaches will always be the largest staple client in any chiropractic practice, and ours is no different. However, we encourage our patients to take a more proactive approach to their healthcare and motivate them to be checked on a more periodic basis, pain or no pain. Despite being a more therapy-oriented practice, we try to de-emphasize pain as an outcome measure. Pain is a signal our body sends to our brain that tells us something isn't quite right. Our body then responds to that signal, sometimes fixing the issue or otherwise creating a more challenging issue. We communicate a simple idea to each patient: the goal is to get to the root cause of the problem so the pain stops on its own. This is also why I do not identify with the straight or mixer classification. Both ends of the spectrum have something to offer patients.

Somewhere in the middle is where most chiropractors fit in today. These types of practices deal with back pain and neck injuries regularly. They also recognize other illnesses, diseases, and everyday ailments can avail care and even be prevented through regular manipulation and adjustment of the spine. To better understand how this type of chiropractor fits into a complete wellness program and integrates with the medical profession, you'll need a better understanding of chiropractic.

Chiropractic Principles and Philosophies

If you were playing soccer, and your opponents were particularly competitive, would you be satisfied playing conservatively for a draw? What has undermined the well-being of our society has been an attitude of suppression versus stimulation. What is this concept of suppression versus stimulation, and what does it mean regarding your healthcare? Would you instead just prevent the other team from scoring, completely ignoring trying to score? Or would you attempt to corral their best offensive player and continue doing your best to put points up?

As a society, we are focused on suppressing the symptom. We focus on getting rid of the cold by taking *something* to knock off the cough or get rid of the headache. We take an antibiotic to get rid of the bacteria that has infected us, creating our ailments. The sad truth is that the more we use the medicine, the more dependent we will become on those medicines to create a normal life.

Suppression alone is not the answer. Our bodies are resilient and have an excellent healing mechanism embedded inside our nervous system. We must learn how to reawaken the power of this healing capacity that we have deep within us all. By focusing on what you want, you can help create the solution to achieve what you want. You don't only want to get rid of this pain; the real goal is to be healthy – which needs stimulation. Those two concepts are radically different, yet people overlook this difference all the time.

We tend to lull ourselves into a false belief that things are just going to get better on their own. Without being proactive, you'll eventually figure out that concept doesn't work either. The sad truth is that 37% of people who die of a heart attack die without a single symptom. The only symptom was death. These are people that just got a check-up, felt fine, got a clean bill of health, and then maybe they went for a run and dropped dead. Something went wrong, and the cause was unknown until the unfortunate happened.

We know that in cancer treatment, if we just focus on suppressing cancer growth without stimulating the body's defensive capacity, we will severely compromise the person's ability to recover from the treatments. Sometimes just the treatment of the disease is what causes the patient to die in the end. This fear is why many cancer patients refuse chemotherapy. Instead, they would try to live out their remaining time on their terms rather than die a crippling death due to the harsh nuclear medicines.

I'm absolutely not trying to put down the medical profession. I know medical doctors do the best they can to provide the best care possible. Cancer and other diabolical diseases are nature's worst creations, and it's heartbreakingly unfair to those suffering. But here's the truth: certain things in our health care system are not working. Medicine should not always be the first and best choice in maintaining health or even treating disease. Even though this is what has been done for generations, it doesn't necessarily mean it is the best method. Chiropractic and other non-allopathic healthcare options started in the first place due to a lack of quality healthcare in medicine. Perhaps this is happening again, especially when we look into the causes of deep-seated issues of over-prescription and opioid addiction.

As we mentioned earlier, there are many terms used in chiropractic that may not be familiar to the layperson; phrases such as *subluxation* or *innate intelligence*. These specific principles are fundamental and form the base of many other theories and practices within chiropractic. This foundation gets detailed further in 33 short statements describing the basis of all chiropractic care. Again, everyone does not adopt these statements, but belongs in the history of our growing, expanding profession.

The 33 Principles of Chiropractic

At some point in their training, all chiropractors learn the 33 Principles. These have become a foundation for chiropractic practice by some and a philosophy by which to live by others. 'The Principles' were authored by a Doctor of Chiropractic, Ralph W. Stephenson, and published in his textbook simply called "Chiropractic Textbook."

As a preface to these 33 concepts, Stephenson stated that they were not the chiropractor's complete and comprehensive rules or beliefs, but a foundation upon which to build. The principles start in a general sense and get increasingly specific. Some chiropractors embrace all of these principles (hence some refer to themselves as "Principled" chiropractors), some do not. That is just one more reason why, as a patient who is seeking healthcare, you will find distinctions between one chiropractor and the next. This is important in finding a chiropractor with whom you feel comfortable and one who shares your philosophy on health.

Here, verbatim, are the 33 Principles of Chiropractic as published by Ralph W. Stephenson, DC in 1927:

1. The Major Premise - A Universal Intelligence is in all matter and continually gives to it all its properties and actions, thus maintaining it in existence.
2. The Chiropractic Meaning of Life - The expression of this intelligence through matter is the Chiropractic meaning of life.
3. The Union of Intelligence and Matter - Life is necessarily the union of intelligence and matter.
4. The Triune of Life - Life is a trinity having three necessary united factors, namely: Intelligence, Force and Matter.
5. The Perfection of the Triune - In order to have 100% Life, there must be 100% Intelligence, 100% Force, 100% Matter.
6. The Principle of Time - There is no process that does not require time.
7. The Amount of Intelligence in Matter - The amount of intelligence for any given amount of matter is 100%, and is always proportional to its requirements.
8. The Function of Intelligence - The function of intelligence is to create force.
9. The Amount of Force Created by Intelligence - The amount of force created by intelligence is always 100%.
10. The Function of Force - The function of force is to unite intelligence and matter.
11. The Character of Universal Forces - The forces of Universal Intelligence are manifested by physical laws; are unswerving

and unadapted, and have no solicitude for the structures in which they work.

12. **Interference with Transmission of Universal Forces** - There can be interference with transmission of universal forces.

13. **The Function of Matter** - The function of matter is to express force.

14. **Universal Life** - Force is manifested by motion in matter; all matter has motion, therefore there is universal life in all matter.

15. **No Motion without the Effort of Force** - Matter can have no motion without the application of force by intelligence.

16. **Intelligence in both Organic and Inorganic Matter** - Universal Intelligence gives force to both organic and inorganic matter.

17. **Cause and Effect** - Every effect has a cause and every cause has effects.

18. **Evidence of Life** - The signs of life are evidence of the intelligence of life.

19. **Organic Matter** - The material of the body of a "living thing" is organized matter.

20. **Innate Intelligence** - A "living thing" has an inborn intelligence within its body, called Innate Intelligence.

21. **The Mission of Innate Intelligence** - The mission of Innate Intelligence is to maintain the material of the body of a "living thing" in active organization.

22. **The Amount of Innate intelligence** - There is 100% of Innate Intelligence in every "living thing," the requisite amount, proportional to its organization.

23. **The Function of Innate Intelligence** - The function of Innate Intelligence is to adapt universal forces and matter for use in

the body, so that all parts of the body will have coordinated action for mutual benefit.

24. The Limits of Adaptation - Innate Intelligence adapts forces and matter for the body as long as it can do so without breaking a universal law, or Innate Intelligence is limited by the limitations of matter.

25. The Character of Innate Forces - The forces of Innate Intelligence never injure or destroy the structures in which they work.

26. Comparison of Universal and Innate Forces - In order to carry on the universal cycle of life, Universal forces are destructive, and Innate forces constructive, as regards structural matter.

27. The Normality of Innate Intelligence - Innate Intelligence is always normal and its function is always normal.

28. The Conductors of Innate Forces - The forces of Innate Intelligence operate through or over the nervous system in animal bodies.

29. Interference with Transmission of Innate Forces - There can be interference with the transmission of innate forces.

30. The Causes of Dis-ease - Interference with the transmission of innate forces causes incoordination of disease.

31. Subluxations - Interference with transmission in the body is always directly or indirectly due to subluxations in the spinal column.

32. The Principle of Coordination - Coordination is the principle of harmonious action of all the parts of an organism, in fulfilling their offices and purposes.

33. The Law of Demand and Supply - The Law of Demand and Supply is existent in the body in its ideal state; wherein the

"clearinghouse," is the brain, Innate the virtuous "banker," brain cells "clerks," and nerve cells "messengers."

Terminology and Glossary

Here we can look at the meaning of some of the key ideas found within chiropractic philosophy. You will also see how they are implemented and applied today. Many will agree Chiropractic is an art (practice), a science (anatomy and physiology), and a philosophy (theory). We delve deeper into the philosophy here. The description of these terms is written with the original language used to explain them and may not be functional in today's practice environment.

Innate Intelligence

The straight chiropractic way of thinking centers on something called "innate intelligence." What this means, in a nutshell, is that the human body is entirely self-sufficient in how it functions. The body automatically knows when to take a breath or increase the heart rate when more oxygen is needed. It sends off a signal when it needs food or water. The body responds to a virus or infection by heating up into a fever to make conditions unlivable for the foreign invader. It does all of this because the brain can automatically send signals to the body without external intervention.

The brain and nervous system as a whole can function whether we are awake or asleep. It knows what it needs and what to do about that need all on its own. The miraculous part of it all is that we are born with this innate intelligence. However, from the beginning, from the process of birth, interference can get in the way of the free flow of the intelligence data needed to make the body perform optimally.

Subluxation

Every organ in the body relies upon innate intelligence to function. Innate intelligence is the force behind the signal from the brain to the body. The blocking of a free-flowing signal from the brain causes problems. It can show up as aches and pains – more alerts that something isn't quite right -- or it can appear over time as illness and disease. This blockage or interference has a name within the straight chiropractic community called "subluxation," or nerve interference. For the chiropractor, the subluxation is synonymous with "dis-ease." Ease is when the signal from the brain to the body flows unimpeded or subluxation-free. A subluxation causes dis-ease, meaning there is a loss of ease in the system. Therefore, subluxation causes a lack of complete function due to the blockage of the signal sent through the nerves.

The spinal column is the primary shield the body has to protect the spinal cord and the nerves. If it is in perfect form and alignment, the messages go about the body unhindered. The body rarely stays in this ideal state. We may "tweak" our backbone doing any number of everyday activities, even during sleep. It could take months or years before any noticeable dis-ease occurs unless there is some major trauma to the spine. Even these seemingly minor misalignments can distort a clear message from transmitting to the muscles or organs it needs to visit. This is subluxation. The cure or solution is to open up that channel once again and let the signals flow freely. This is what chiropractic is all about.

An application to this idea of subluxation is stress. Stress can cause several issues, but typically, within the philosophy, subluxation is further subdivided into emotional, physical, or chemical stress. Subluxation in a broader sense can refer not just to nerve signals and messages but any disruption of any spinal joint's function or physical stress. Either physical or emotional stress can cause chemical stress by wreaking havoc with our hormonal balances. Cortisol, a hormone secreted by our adrenal glands, is one of the central players in these types of subluxations. Emotional stress caused by mental turmoil can have physical and chemical effects. What our brain feels, our body makes real.

The only known way to correct a subluxation is to get a chiropractic adjustment. Chiropractors train to remove any nerve interference through the gentle application of force to specific areas of the spine.

Depending on the chiropractor you work with, there can be slightly different interpretations of a subluxation; some may not even believe it exists. Many researchers have attempted to establish a scientific theory of the "Vertebral Subluxation Complex" or "VSC," but the scientific evidence has yet to bear robust findings. As such, subluxation remains a philosophical point of division within the profession.

"Subluxation deniers," evidence-based chiropractors, or mixers typically go with the word 'restriction' to avoid being embroiled in a century-long debate over terminology. Typically, mixers explain the origin of the issue similarly, omitting generalizations the subluxation concept offers. Simply put, mixers refer to an improperly moving segment or joint as a restriction and either use an adjustment or manipulation to restore proper function. Whether the practitioner acknowledges the neurological benefit of that specific maneuver is subject to personal philosophy.

A Self-Check

You can examine yourself monthly to check for signs that you might require an adjustment. These simple exercises, 11 in all, are safe for the entire family, even young children. Any test that you cannot perform should act as an alarm, indicating that you need to examine the area further. The tests focus on range of motion, posture, and leg length. With each test, you rate yourself as having "normal," "restricted," or "painful" results. On the leg length test, you will periodically check to see if your legs are equal in length or if the right or left leg is shorter than the other. As a rule, never force any movements beyond your comfort level.

11 Self Tests for Spinal Restriction

Range of Motion

Perform these tests while standing and in a relaxed position.

1. Rotation -- Turn your head slowly to the right, then to the left. Do not move your upper body. You should be able to turn so that your chin is nearly parallel with your shoulder.

2. Lateral Flexion – Tilt your head slowly to the right and then left, keeping your shoulders relaxed. You should be able to bring your ears to within a couple of inches from the shoulders.

3. Flexion/Extension – Bend your head to the front and then back slowly. Look straight down and then all the way up.

4. Waist Rotation – Keeping your head in line with the upper body, turn to the left and right from the hips. You should be able to rotate approximately 45 degrees in each direction.

5. Lateral Flexion – Standing straight, bend to the side from the waist 45 degrees to the left and then the right. Slide your hand down the side of your thigh to your knee.

6. Flexion/Extension – Keeping the back and legs straight, bend from the waist forward, then backward. You should be able to bend forward at a 90-degree angle and, when leaning back, be able to look straight above you.

Postural Checks

Do these tests standing in front of a full-length mirror. You will want to take a few deep breaths and try to relax before examining your posture in the mirror.

7. Midline – Imagine a vertical line that runs straight down your body. It runs from the head, through the nose and chin, right down through the navel to your feet. Compare it to a vertical line on the mirror's edge to see if the two are parallel.

8. Ears – Imagine a horizontal line that runs from ear to ear through the middle of your head. Then compare it to the horizontal line on the edge of the mirror. These two lines should be parallel too.

9. Shoulders – Imagine a horizontal line now from shoulder to shoulder. Compare it to the horizontal line of the mirror's edge. These two lines should be parallel as well.

10. Hips -- Finally, do the same horizontal check at the hip level. Imagine the horizontal line from hip to hip, or touch your hips with both hands, and compare it to the mirror's edge to see if the two are parallel.

Leg Length Check

This test requires a partner. The person being tested lies on his or her back on a flat, firm surface, usually the floor. The partner checks the heels of your feet with the fingers outside and thumbs pressing gently on the heels. Judging by the location of one thumb compared to the other, the partner may see a slightly shorter leg on one side.

After doing each test at home, you will have valuable information to give to the chiropractor. This monthly self-exam can also track any changes that could indicate a subluxation or joint restriction. It may help evaluate if you are engaging in any activities that may be inviting problems for your spine.

Chiropractic Care for Restrictions of the Spine

The role of chiropractic is to find and correct restrictions in the spine. There are a few different ways that chiropractors go about doing this. The "old-fashioned" way is still one of the best methods for detecting misalignment of the spine. Through hands-on techniques, chiropractors feel for misaligned vertebrae blocking signals from the brain to the body. Chiropractors are known for a highly developed sense of touch. Years of hands-on clinical training enable him or her to feel for misalignments that could be blocking the free flow of nerve signals. However, even as well developed as this unique sense of touch is, chiropractors today also rely on many other medical devices and advances in medical technology to help create an even more complete picture of what is happening within the body.

A popular method of creating an image of the spine is through X-ray. All chiropractic colleges have extensive coursework and practical experience in interpreting X-rays. The two methods used together give the Doctor of Chiropractic an excellent overall picture of the spinal situation for the patient. Some chiropractors have the provisions to take the x-ray in their facility, and others refer out. Some advanced techniques require a regular x-ray to be taken to track spinal changes. Although this has been a traditional method of assessing patients, chiropractic regulatory bodies have tightened up policy and procedure regarding x-rays. Typically, trauma or suspicion of osteoporosis or fracture requires x-ray examination.

Some cases are easier to locate the spinal origin than others. For example, if a patient comes to the office complaining of pain shooting down their leg, it is relatively easy to locate the vertebra, which is probably causing the "pinched" nerve. In reality, it may be that there are several vertebrae misaligned, and only the one responsible for protecting nerves to the legs is pressing on the actual nerve. Another possibility could be that the intervertebral disc, a sturdy piece of cartilage between spinal bones, has bulged outwardly, applying physical pressure on a delicate spinal nerve.

In other situations, the spinal restriction may not be as apparent to the average person, but it is to the chiropractor. Each vertebra in the spinal column has a bundle of nerves that protrude. Each nerve - the wire that sends and receives messages - is appointed to a different organ or system in the body. So, if a patient comes into the office complaining of chronic stomach aches, then it may be the nerves coming from the mid-back are being blocked in some way by the vertebrae intended to protect them. Evaluation and treatment can result in a faster resolution since the adjustment addresses the cause of the problem.

Dr. R.L. Hartman developed a spinal nerve chart (sometimes referred to as a Meric Chart) that shows the effects of specific vertebral dysfunction on various systems and organs in the body. The table here summarizes and outlines some of the conditions or ailments that could result from pinched nerves or areas of restriction. It is not a final diagnostic 'subluxation finder,' but it is a good tool for examining which nerves may be affected by spinal changes. It helps the chiropractor know where to start after listening to the patient's complete history, including any symptoms they are experiencing.

Corresponding Vertebrae & Nerves to Symptoms & Conditions *

Vertebra	Parts of the Body Related to Corresponding Nerves	Symptoms or Conditions Possibly Resulting from Subluxation/Restriction
Cervical Spine		
C1	head, brain, face, pituitary gland, inner and middle ear, blood flow to this region	headaches, mental conditions, nervousness, dizziness, high blood pressure
C2	eyes, sinuses, auditory and optical nerves, tongue, forehead	sinus and allergy problems, deafness, blindness
C3	face bones, teeth	acne, eczema
C4	nose, mouth, mucous membranes	hay fever, post-nasal drip, infections in adenoids
C5	neck glands and vocal cords	sore throats and laryngitis
C6	muscles and glands in the neck, tonsils	tonsillitis, cough, croup, pain in the neck and upper arm
C7	thyroid gland, elbows	bursitis, tendonitis, over or underactive thyroid

Thoracic Spine		
T1	forearms, wrists, hands, fingers	pain in these regions and breathing problems, asthma
T2	heart valves and coronary arteries	heart conditions and chest pain
T3	lungs, chest, breast	bronchitis, pneumonia, congestion
T4	gal bladder	all conditions of the gall bladder, including jaundice, shingles
T5	liver, blood	liver conditions, low blood pressure, arthritis, anemia
T6	stomach	gastrointestinal problems, heartburn, indigestion
T7	pancreas	diabetes and hypoglycemia
T8	spleen and diaphragm	serious infections and hic-ups
T9	adrenal glands	anemia, hair loss, obesity, allergies
T10	kidneys	fatigue, kidney malfunction
T11	kidneys and urethras	skin conditions
T12	lymph nodes, fallopian tubes, small intestines	rheumatism, infertility, gas pains

L1	large intestines, colon	diarrhea, constipation, hernias, colitis
L2	appendix, upper leg	appendicitis, varicose veins
L3	ovaries, uterus, testicles, bladder, knee	menstrual problems, impotence, bed wetting, knee pain
L4	prostate, lower back, sciatic nerve	painful or frequent urination, sciatica, backaches
L5	lower legs, ankles, feet, toes	poor circulation, leg cramps, foot and ankle swelling and pain
Sacrum	hips, buttocks	spinal curvatures
Coccyx	rectum, anus	hemorrhoids, pain while sitting

*Table is only a partial listing and summarization of items contained on Dr. Hartman's Spinal Nerve Chart.

Chapter 8

The Spine

The primary component of chiropractic is, of course, the spine. For the sake of our discussion, the spine, which contains the spinal cord, vertebrae, and intervertebral discs, is central to chiropractic science. Giving you a little anatomy lesson on the spine will help you understand how and why chiropractic makes so much sense to those who have adopted this practice as our lifelong vocation.

The spinal column is a row of bones that encircle the spinal cord. The spinal cord is the conduit component of the central nervous system, which transmits signals throughout the body, to and from the brain. Some people assume that the spinal cord and nerves only transmit signals about touch and pain, which is far from the truth.

In simple terms, the nerves signal the brain when you touch something hot, pain then registers in the brain, and you quickly remove your hand from the heat. Outside of that single function, the nervous system communicates much more information to the brain and other organs in the body.

Nerves supply every area of the body with information, either from the brain or another area of the body. When there is no interference (what some chiropractors refer to as subluxation or restriction) in the message transmitted, every nerve can supply its target at its maximum capacity. A target is usually a group of cells (tissue) or organized tissues (organ). That is the number one purpose of chiropractic – to remove static from the message signals and open the channels for the body to mend and heal using its built-in ability to heal.

Regions of the Spine

The spine divides into three key regions. The first seven bones of the neck, starting from the base of the skull, are referred to as the cervical spine. Twelve bones of the thoracic spine (mid-back) follow and finally end with five bones in the lumbar spine or low back. There is also a fourth area referred to as the sacrum, which used to be four separate bones but fused through the evolutionary process. Just below the sacrum is the tiny coccyx or tailbone, which is actually a vestigial or redundant remnant of when human beings had tails! The sacrum and coccyx are at the bottom of the spine and extend into the pelvic area.

Within the three central regions of the spine, the vertebrae are all assigned numbers. In misalignments or restrictions of a particular vertebra, the chiropractor may explain that the issue is coming from the 'C4 vertebra,' for example. This listing means that the 4th vertebra from the *top*, or the *4th* vertebra in the *Cervical* spine, is misaligned or restricted.

A patient who has a blockage or misalignment in the C4 vertebra could be seeing the doctor about their hay fever and not necessarily neck pain. That is because the nerves that extend from the C4 vertebra are responsible for messages sent to the nose, lips, mouth, eustachian tube, and mucous membranes. Often, a misalignment here manifests itself as hay fever, postnasal drip, adenoid infections, or other upper respiratory symptoms. Although further study to scientifically conclude these connections requires to be done, enough case report data exists to suggest some cause and effect between adjustment of this area and alleviation of reported symptoms.

Every nerve that extends from the spinal column is responsible for an organ, function, or performance of some part of the body. This includes essential organs such as those that provide sensory capabilities of touch, found in every anatomical area. A complete body map shows this radial effect. Envision an outline of the body and extend lines from the center where the spine would be located, drawn out to each extremity. This illustration roughly shows how the nerves and vertebrae provide signal coverage to those areas within the body. Since the vertebral column protects each nerve, you can now see how even slight spinal misalignments can wreak havoc on the whole body.

This idea of labeling vertebrae and their corresponding nerves is not exclusive to chiropractic. The medical field also recognizes the anatomy and what it means to have something out of alignment. Mainstream medicine and chiropractic differ in how spinal misalignment is treated and assessing the misalignment's full impact. The term *subluxation* in medical speak means a joint's physical dislocation, where chiropractic means a minor misalignment, specifically of a spinal segment.

How the Spine Moves

The spine has an unusual shape. If one were to look at a typical, healthy spine flush from behind, one would see a neat row of bones in a straight line. But view the same healthy spine from the side, and you would see three distinct curves. The cervical spine and the lumbar spine (the top and bottom) are called "lordosis" and curve forward (the convex side of the curve faces forward). The thoracic spine creates a "kyphosis" and curves the opposite way (the convex side of the curve faces backward). So, if you looked at a typical, healthy spine from the side, you might see an "S" curve, which is entirely normal.

The spine can bend, move and return to its "s"-like shape without incident or injury because of soft tissue that works together with the bony vertebrae. Two features are essential in helping the spinal column protect the large central nerve - the spinal cord.

The first feature - an intervertebral disc - can be found between each vertebra. This thick piece of cartilage helps absorb shock as the spine bends and twists during normal movement and activity. It also protects the vertebrae and spine from excessive shock. You don't think about these details as you bend down to pick up a toy off the floor because everything is in its proper place. You can even bend and twist to one side to grasp the toy that slid under the chair. Still no problems. However, discs do break down, despite being there for the nerve's protection. Deterioration or slight deformation of that disc could cause pinching of a nerve, leading to pain.

This type of back injury or painful condition is among the most common reasons people visit a chiropractor. Luckily, this is one of the issues chiropractic has an impressive and well-documented track record with, so most people that start with disc injuries leave with no pain. Once the disc issue resolves, participating in some preventive care is essential.

The second spinal feature that helps in protecting the nerve is the facet joint. The shape of the facet joint allows for limited movement of the spine. These joints are oriented differently in the cervical, thoracic, and lumbar spine. They regulate the joint's range of motion, so routine movements cannot injure the spinal cord. This orientation allows most rotation to occur in the cervical region, most side bending to occur in the thoracic spine, and most forward and backward bending in the lumbar spine.

With its built-in ability to heal, the body was created in a way that protects the most vital organs. The ribs protect the heart and lungs. The skull protects the brain. The spinal column protects the spinal cord. The body's design is intricate and elegant!

Misaligned Vertebrae

Every nerve in the body that originates from the spinal cord supplies critical information to the area of the body for which it is responsible. The example of the C4 vertebra being out of alignment is just one of the hundreds of slight misalignments that can cause interference with the nerve signal and result in an ailment. From the spinal cord, 31 pairs of spinal nerve roots extend out at every level of the spine, including the sacrum and coccyx. These 62 nerve roots branch exponentially to give rise to the astonishing number of 7 trillion nerves and nerve endings throughout the entire body!

A patient visiting a medical doctor for indigestion or heartburn will almost immediately receive a prescription for some kind of antacid to ease those uncomfortable symptoms. For some people, this kind of quick fix may be okay for a while. After all, we want to get rid of painful discomfort as quickly as possible. The problem with this treatment is that it doesn't cure the problem. It very superficially addresses the issue and indeed neglects the real cause of the problem. How can the body ever hope to heal itself if medications are momentarily quieting the symptoms?

Symptoms are present for a reason. The body, in its wisdom, has to let the brain know something isn't right. If we quiet that signal with medication, it's like telling someone to stop talking while trying to warn you about impending danger. They are trying to give you an important message, but you will eventually have to deal with a much bigger problem if you ignore it long enough.

When there is a symptom related to the stomach, it can often arise from the T6 vertebra. It is from this area that stomach problems and the body's ability to correct them transmit. The nerves in the T6 region could be experiencing some kind of interference. Removing that blockage through an adjustment of the spine will open up the lines of communication to the stomach and allow the problems in that region to be corrected naturally. With such few nerves emerging from the spinal cord, even small amounts of pressure can have far-reaching implications.

This simplified lesson on the anatomy of the spine illustrates the complex nature of the spinal column and the central nervous system. It is not quite as simple as explained here. Many minor misalignments exist that can impact a single region of the body. Likewise, there are many different ways in which symptoms manifest themselves that it isn't always easy to pinpoint just what the real problem is. Examining the issue from multiple angles is often required and sometimes the opposite of what mainstream medical care offers. The ability to think outside of the box is one area in which chiropractors excel.

Back pain can often originate in the stomach and vice versa. Headaches can be the symptom of many other ailments that may start in a completely different body area. The complexities of this whole system are what chiropractors study for years to perform the proper diagnostic tests and begin the correct treatment for any specific ailment.

Chapter 9

Spinal Manipulations and Adjustments

After the diagnostic stage of a visit to the chiropractor, there is the treatment phase of patient care. This is the moment you've been waiting for - the hands-on physical part of the chiropractic visit. There is one final diagnostic stage before any actual spinal manipulation or adjustment, which is spinal palpation. Palpation is a hands-on maneuver using touch to determine changes or irregularities in tissues along the spine.

Spinal palpation can be either static or using motion. In static palpation, the chiropractor examines the muscles and joints using touch while the patient is still. Primarily, this process tests for sensitivity or pain and can detect swelling. Motion palpation allows the chiropractor to measure joint motion with touch. Chiropractors move joints to the very end range of their physiological limit, referred to as 'end play.' The degree of end play, with or without pain, is a useful diagnostic piece of data to have before any adjustments.

Manipulations to Remove Joint Restrictions

Manipulating the spine through small, gentle movements of the vertebrae is the most effective way of eliminating restrictions of the spine. Limitations of the spine can prevent the nerves from sending a clear, uninterrupted signal from the spinal column, leading to illness and disease over time. Chiropractors employ what is known as a "high velocity, low amplitude" (HVLA) thrust over a joint to remove the restriction at that joint. This maneuver is known as a chiropractic adjustment or manipulation.

In straight chiropractic, the term 'disease' breaks down to 'dis-ease.' This implies a reduction in wellness, instead of the medical word, which means more chronic or life-threatening illness. There is a fine distinction, but with chiropractic, the ideas of the body being seen as a whole and restoring its full functionality are central to allowing the body to be the best it can be. This state of being returned to a wholly healthy and balanced state is known as "homeostasis."

That Cracking Sound

The images of Rambo jumping out of the bushes and twisting a bad guy's neck, *CRACK!* The baddie's head turns to an unnatural position, and he very slowly slumps to the ground, quite obviously dead. This depiction is what most people fear when visiting a chiropractor. Even though the bones are being gently adjusted and the movement is safe, some people just hate the noise it makes. The "popping" sound many people hear during an adjustment is called "cavitation."

Cavitation occurs from within the joint capsule. Imagine a hinge that is just not moving correctly. A couple of squeezes from the oil can, and the door opens and closes like a charm. Every joint in the spine has a sac-like covering called the joint capsule. Within the sac is a very slippery lubricant called synovial fluid. The sound made by cavitation is the release of nitrogen gases from the synovial fluid in the joint and is painless. It is a reaction that allows the joint surfaces to slide freely over each other, thereby reducing restriction.

Types of Adjustments

Spinal adjustment in the early days of chiropractic involved almost all hands-on movement of the vertebrae to release the restriction in the spine. The amount of pressure, angle of the maneuver, and position of the hands are the primary methods for varying the effects of the adjustment.

Today during an adjustment, misalignments are corrected through both hands-on techniques and the use of instruments. Both methods are effective in their primary objective: to return vertebrae to their proper positions and function. Most chiropractors today use many different techniques to realign the vertebrae. Some are done strictly by hand, while others employ such instruments as an activator, a rubber-tipped handheld instrument. The following discussion lists some of the more common techniques. There are over 200 techniques that chiropractors can learn and use in clinical practice.

Adjustments in children are different than for adults. The smaller and still developing bones require a much lighter touch. Chiropractors can perform these adjustments with either one hand or just a few fingers. Manipulations using gentle fingertip pressure are done even on infants just a few minutes old.

Applied Kinesiology

Kinesiology focuses on the muscles around the bones as well as the vertebrae themselves. Special procedures balance the muscles related to the specific vertebrae. Adjustments of the spine stay in place longer when the attached muscles are performing optimally. A series of muscle tests are carried out before any manipulations and frequently re-checked through the treatment.

Table Adjustments

Adjustments on a chiropractic table may be the most familiar technique, even to those new to chiropractic. During a table adjustment, the patient lies down on a specialized table. The chiropractor applies quick thrusts to specific areas of the spine. Simultaneous with the thrust, the table drops slightly, with a mechanism built into the table called a gravity assist. This little feature is handy for various ailments and parts of the body and can suit different issues by altering the tension for the drop piece. This is a gentler method than the straight manual adjustment. Less pressure is needed to get the spine to move and is sometimes the preferred method for certain sensitive conditions.

Toggle Drop

A toggle drop also uses quick thrusts. The hands are crossed and applied to the problem point on the spine. It is a method that is highly effective in improving vertebral joint mobility. This is also one of the more ancient techniques in chiropractic lore.

Lumbar Roll

With the lumbar roll, a patient lies on their side. The result effectively focuses on one specific vertebra out of alignment in the low back and pelvic region. Interestingly, this technique is also helpful in a general sense and can apply changes to an extensive spinal range. Again, quick thrusts are the primary mobilizing factor to restricted segments.

Instrumental Adjustments

An instrument adjustment begins with the patient lying face down on the table. A spring-loaded instrument is used to provide a very gentle movement of the vertebrae. This technique is gentle enough for children, the elderly, overly sensitive tissues, and small joints. This instrument technique is highly adaptable and can be used for many hard-to-access body landmarks.

Chapter 10

Phases of Healing

In the previous chapter, we have explained how chiropractic practices aid in returning your system to a healthy, optimal state. To better comprehend how this approach can help with increasing your strength, health, and longevity, this section will discuss the specific cycles of chiropractic healing. But before we jump onto this, we need to re-affirm this statement - chiropractic care isn't a fast cure or overnight miracle. If your system is decidedly out of whack, it is due to years of built-up, unresolved issues. While the good news is that it won't take years to regain your health, it will take some dedicated amount of time for the body to heal. Therefore, you need to practice patience and consistency. Let's delve deeper into the cycles, which should help make sense of where you might be on this spectrum.

Stage 1: The Intense Inflammatory Phase

Inflammation is a lot like contending with a hotly burning fire. This is the stage that urges people to pay more attention and seek some type of expert help. The interventions pursued could be conventional medical methods or alternative means, the latter usually when prescription drugs do not achieve the desired effects. Why is that? During the inflammation stage, the symptoms are hot and not quickly subdued. The best bet to combat this blaze is to find the source.

Remember previously in this book where we pointed out the misconception that chiropractic practice was painful? Chiropractic methods in their basic form are not painful. Pain is triggered when pain sensors, called *nociceptors,* are disturbed or activated by some form of damage. These specialized cells then relay the signals to the somatosensory region of your brain. From here, the brain can send corresponding messages telling the body how it should react. In a simplistic example, seeking shade on a hot day is a response to a disturbance. Removing the body from a damaging environment is one of the easiest ways to avoid further harm. In some cases, the answer to tissue damage is to tighten up the muscles surrounding the area of concern, walling it off to protect the area.

Prolonged exposure to the pain stimulus (or cause of pain) can create a ratcheting effect, where the system runs through this process several times, creating tighter and tighter muscles. Eventually, increasingly more minor stimuli will cause the entire system to trigger unnecessarily strong responses, which experts call *hypersensitivity* to pain.

In this stage, outside of pain, the patient may also experience discomfort like swelling, itchiness, redness, or loss of balance. Patients who come to visit us in this stage are not doing so because they want to improve their health, but they are overwhelmed with pain. Their main concern is to reduce their pain and symptoms and not the underlying mechanisms or origins of their issue.

Pain is a profoundly subjective experience, which necessarily remains unique to the individual. Researchers continue to look for common traits among acute pain sufferers; however, conclusive evidence about what triggers painful episodes remains out of reach. Some factors that influence pain include:

Sex

Age

Height

Weight

Chronicity of pain (how long pain has been present)

Compliance to prescription (how well you follow the doctor's directions)

Pain tolerance level

Co-morbidities (other health problems)

Upon the initial consultation, the chiropractor will assess all the above parameters and any other relevant issues to develop a personalized plan for your case. They will document your specific needs and challenges and incorporate them into your schedule. However, this isn't like medicine--the chiropractic approach isn't the same for everyone. Similar conditions may be treated with similar treatment, but every treatment is tailor-made for the individual.

Stage 2: The Restorative And Corrective Stage

During this stage, pain and discomfort begin to subside. Your pain will become much more tolerable, and while you won't feel as if you are running like a world-class athlete, you will most likely feel better and have a more positive mood. For example, sitting or standing may no longer be painful.

Here, we rely on rehabilitation, gaining strength, and repairing damaged tissues' integrity, which aids the road to full recovery. This is a positive stage for everybody involved, as the patient starts to feel better. The energy levels of the patient begin to increase, and the range of motion is restored. Pain "eats" vast amounts of energy, so any reduction of pain automatically confers rest. Many chronic pain patients may also suffer from chronic fatigue for this reason alone. The mental stress of being in pain for so long creates fatigue, physically and mentally. Once that cycle of pain breaks, it's like a spell lifts, and the patient feels energy coursing through their body.

It is precisely at this juncture that the patient should exercise additional caution. Despite the sudden ability to perform long-avoided actions, patients must avoid pushing and forcing that movement too early. The issue is, if you go too hard, tissues that are still healing may become dysfunctional. Think of a cut in the skin that is just beginning to heal. If you pick the scab before it fully forms, the laceration will most likely reopen and begin to bleed again. We want to avoid this for the healing muscle and joint soft tissue, so make sure to follow instructions as closely as possible and avoid getting too excited! As mentioned earlier, pain is usually the first thing that shows up, and usually the first thing to go away once treatment begins. The danger is that the underlying issue may still be lurking around somewhere and must not reaggravate.

During this phase, our aim with chiropractic treatment is to coordinate our movements to improved spinal mobility so that your spine and nerves return to healthy physiological function. Depending on the severity of your condition, you may still need to attend follow-up visits each week as treatment continues to solidify and heal the injured structures. Though each treatment plan varies from professional to professional, one standard piece of advice given throughout the rehabilitation world is to continue doing the most demanding work you can painlessly—taking risks with new challenges can wait.

Keep in mind that this correcting stage tends to be the longest one. Other limitations and factors can surely affect the speed of the healing progress, both positively and negatively. The severity of the issue, for example, could dictate the length of this stage. Imagine the difference between a patient visiting the clinic after a severe car accident and a patient with problems stemming from a night of poor sleeping posture. In the car accident victim's case, we can expect a longer treatment duration in this stage. Some other things that affect the therapy length or create a slower healing process are:

Poor diet/nutrition

Smoking

Stress

Improper ergonomics

A negative mindset

The opposite of this is also true! If you're a non-smoker with a healthy, balanced diet, who takes care of your stress and remains optimistic about your outcome (yes, such a person does exist!), we can expect a faster than average restoration process. Even if you make positive inroads in any one of these areas, we can see an improvement in your outcome sooner. That's how efficiently your body can work while under Chiropractic care. It's well-documented that adjustments to the spine lower stress and improve poor ergonomics. So, the treatment you get in this stage kickstarts a healthy change in your lifestyle as well.

Stage 3: The Maintenance Stage

I'll be honest here - I love seeing a patient get to this specific stage in their healing. Getting to this stage means that they have followed the treatment plan and are doing what they can to prioritize their health. Patients in this stage often report that they feel the best they have ever felt - maybe in their entire life. The pain is under control, minimized, or completely gone, to a point where it's almost forgotten. I say 'almost' forgotten because patients often opt to undergo maintenance or wellness care to never return to their state of ill health. The grim reminder of their suffering is also their motivation to stay healthy!

Once the system achieves a state of health, it is necessary to maintain it. The good thing is that it's much easier to maintain this healthy status while you go through this phase. Remember that optimal health doesn't only imply a lack of pain and disease – it is a state of ideal physical, mental, and even interpersonal well-being. This difference is more than an average oil change – this is a lifestyle change!

Another advantage is that even if an injury again hampers you, it will recover more quickly in this state of health. Being in maintenance mode also means you won't need an extended, arduous treatment plan for recovery afterward. Consider this: when a highly practiced and fit athlete endures an injury, he/she recovers more quickly than the average Joe (provided that the athlete doesn't push their limits too far and use the injured part more than they should). The athlete is used to conditioning practices, and their systems are already in optimal health. Recovery, for this reason, is much faster. Trainers often call this 'muscle memory' - the ability for your muscles and joints to "remember" what being in the proper position feels like and automatically default to the correct position.

Consider children and the rate at which they recover from biomechanical injuries. This is because our systems are wired from a very young age to recover and restore perfect health. As we grow older, though, the recovery rate starts to slow down. We are less resistant to strain and cannot fight health problems as quickly as younger people. However, during the maintenance stage, the system is re-loaded with healing capacity, the body works more optimally than before, making healing far easier.

Maintenance goes deeper than a periodic chiropractic session. It boils down to lifetime habits and patterns. A slight increase in stress may occur at this juncture, as this wellness lifestyle translates to additional daily effort. Along with a healthy spine, there are now considerations to be given towards a nutritious diet, exercise, and a positive, stress-free mindset.

In this line of work, we have heard every excuse in the book on why a patient's wellness plan falls flat and pain returns. I'll be the first to tell you that I have probably used all the same excuses! I'm a human being too! The most widely used excuse – by a large margin - is a lack of sufficient time. Face it, we all have time. We all have the same 24 hours every day. Yes, it's true; some people have different priorities, and therein lies the catch. Planning is essential if you're one of the chronically bogged down types, so managing your time should be your primary focus. If everything is well planned, leaving some buffer for unexpected events, things can work to your advantage. The prioritizing of your health means that you will then be able to take care of everyone who leans on you, to the fullest extent possible.

Nathaniel Branden, an inspiring psychologist who has authored many books about self-confidence and self-esteem, has a thought-provoking take on the rationale for priorities. He states that the things we try to improve are the things we already realize. The areas that we neglect to work on are those that we ignore. Some may even believe these neglected areas are beyond our control.

The prioritization rationale also applies to our health. If you don't realize that your eating habits make you gain weight, you won't work on them. Hence it becomes an issue that is out of our control. Good health doesn't occur overnight; you must work on it every day. When options appear on how your health may improve, recognize them, especially when coming from a health expert. Once you realize the issue, prioritize it and then work towards improving it—problem to solution, in three easy steps.

Let's make it even easier. Ask yourself these questions:

Why do I have to eat nutritiously?

Why should I exercise today?

Then:

What foods can I eat that are healthy and taste delicious?

What type of exercise or activity can I do that I enjoy?

And finally:

How can I enjoy today by eating well and exercising?

The 9 Key Habits Of Healthy Folks

Now that you are familiar with the stages of chiropractic science, we can jump to the nine essential habits that healthy folks practice daily, which are vital for good health. This information will help you make more thoughtful and life-changing decisions.

These nine habits trigger substantial lifestyle adjustments, one step at a time. Like in the case of every new change, if you push it too aggressively too soon, you will most likely burn out and come up with the excuse later that "it just didn't work out" and avoid making another attempt. Here are the fundamental principles.

1. Water/Hydration

Every day we'll joyously sip our cup of coffee or can of soda. But when it comes to drinking a glass of water, we tend to brush it off. Most people just can't force themselves to drink it that easy. But drinking plain water is vital for our health—after all, 95% of our systems are water-based - not coffee or a fizzy drink. Furthermore, water can help expel toxins from our systems. Various studies have confirmed that drinking at least eight glasses of water daily can substantially impact the system's power to preserve health and fight off disorders.

2. Vegetables

Kids hate vegetables. But our parents weren't wrong when they forced us to eat our veggies, especially green ones full of vitamins like spinach and broccoli. Increasing your daily consumption of greens is one of the wisest nutritional decisions you can make for your health. Consider this from a scientific perspective. When vegetables are out in nature, they convert light into energy, a process called photosynthesis. By consuming whole, raw, green leafy vegetables, you benefit from the same energy from the sun.

Not all your vegetables need to be eaten raw, but evidence suggests that most raw vegetables contain far more nutritional value than cooked. Cooking vegetables denatures some of the healthier elements held in the vegetable's constitution, like minerals and proteins, which decreases their nutritional value overall. Despite making them more palatable in some instances, you might do better to increase the amount of raw vegetables you eat.

3. Antioxidants

Antioxidants are the key defenders against the effects of destructive free radicals. Free radicals spring from bad cell reactions, which accumulate as we age. Excessive free radicals cause cancer, according to some studies. However, free radicals arise by more than the aging process. Other factors like stress, injuries, or a diet laden with processed and chemically loaded foods are also to blame for creating free radicals.

Our parents would always tell us to eat our fruits and veggies, and they had a very valid reason for doing so. One of the best reasons to eat them is that they are naturally abundant in antioxidants. Mary Beth Russell, registered dietician, explains that antioxidants are essential nutrients that you consume from your food that police cell function. These molecules ensure the proper operation of cellular reactions that are supposed to happen inside your system, thereby preventing the creation of free radicals.

An abundance of antioxidants in your system makes it more capable of fighting and eradicating inflammatory ailments like cardiovascular disease, diabetes, irritable bowel syndrome, and even cancer. Antioxidants are not scarce to find - they are in fruits, veggies, tea, and even wine. A basic thumb rule is that the more vivid color a fruit or veggie has, the more antioxidants they most likely contain. So how many antioxidants should we consume daily? Experts say five portions of fruits or veggies per day. This is an easy addition to your diet that will pay off for years to come.

4. Healthy Oils

Not all fats are considered equal! Oils and fats are an essential part of our metabolism, even though the mainstream media has vilified things like cholesterol in recent times. Contrary to popular belief, eating fat does not make you fat! Let me further clarify that - eating the right fats does not make you fat. Many people lack certain fatty acids, molecules that makeup fats and oils, that could benefit our health. Based on studies, the average person can be lacking up to 90% of vital fatty acids! Insufficient essential fatty acid intake relates to heart and brain diseases, among many other inflammatory disorders. Now, don't swallow that bottle of vegetable oil in your cabinet; it doesn't work like that. Only certain oils are healthy, specifically unsaturated fats and omega-three fatty acids. The avoid list includes saturated fats and trans fats.

5. Proper oxygenation

It is vital to repeatedly allow proper oxygenation of the tissues through mindful breathing methods (cardiovascular exercise can help you out here). Very few of us know how to breathe correctly, and even fewer of us practice proper breathing techniques. Deep, slow breathing throughout the day can help regulate stress, improve mental clarity, boost muscle function, and improve mood!

6. Good Posture

A good reason we cannot breathe correctly is that we have less than adequate posture. When we stand or sit, with our shoulders drawn forward or hunched up, we place strain on our breathing canals, including our diaphragm and lungs. Bad posture additionally puts stress on the spinal curve, and this creates issues with the nervous system. It can also play a significant role in our moods as well.

7. Physical activity and exercise

Yep, we know that this is challenging, and we all come up with various excuses not to get ourselves moving. But whether you like it or not, exercise and physical activity, in general, is vital for your health. There are no acceptable excuses such as babysitting, running around doing house chores, or being too busy. Your system needs a complete plan that activates a vital muscle in your system - the heart. You have to challenge it positively to get it moving more blood and oxygen throughout your body. The more you can challenge it healthily, the better it will work for your system.

8. Adequate sleep

It's no surprise that Indians lack enough sleep every night. India's own Prime Minister, Narendra Modi, is famous for his minuscule sleeping habits, reportedly sleeping only 4 hours every day. While it may look like it works for him and allows him to be super productive, the research about sleep tells us the opposite story.

The hard truth is that most adults will require 6-8 hours of sleep every day for optimal cognitive function. The issue is that insufficient sleep is a sneaky culprit for poor health. People who don't sleep enough have a higher risk of suffering from low immune system function. So, besides inducing tiredness and fatigue, lack of sleep can also lead to the onset of other issues due to suppressed immunity. We heal in our sleep. Sleeping allows stress to decrease and allows our tissues to recuperate.

Sleep deficit disorder is a genuine problem and affects millions worldwide. The systemic loss of adequate amounts of sleep surreptitiously leeches strength and stamina from our bodies before we end up having a crash – a sudden onset of uncontrollable fatigue. And contrary to popular belief, there is no way to catch up on sleep! Simply sleeping an extra 2 or 3 hours on weekends does not bring you back up to speed on the lost sleep during the week. Lifestyle changes are a must in these cases.

9. Positive mindset

We don't want to sound like we have our heads in the clouds or promote esoteric stuff, but there is a point in having a positive mindset. The famous phrase "don't cry over spilled milk" is appropriate here. Yes, it's unfortunate that the milk has spilled, but there's no point dwelling on it since we cannot reverse this event. Mindfulness is the practice of staying present in the here and now. Practicing being grateful, only worrying about the things you can control, and even prayer or spirituality practice go a long way in developing and maintaining a positive mindset.

Let's say you catch a cold, and you moan and complain about it. You will certainly end up feeling worse. But if you work with it instead of "cursing it' and don't pay it much attention, you'll recover faster, almost magically. Of course, this doesn't imply that you should go kickboxing or run five kilometers when you are ill. This is a signal that maybe your system needs some rest, so take a break.

By practicing these nine lifestyle habits and believing in them, you will manifest a healthier reality for yourself. In the following sections, we are going to explain each of these in more detail.

Chapter 11

Healthy Organs

This chapter will explore the major systems in the body and how they should behave optimally for total health. It's a brief overview, and indeed there are deep and far spread complications that can affect organ function, farther than the scope of this book. I hope to provide some basic knowledge of the essential anatomy and connect it back to how chiropractic can benefit all this marvelous machinery!

The Heart

How is the heart such a miraculous muscle? Synchronicity could be a way of describing the heart. It is an elaborate pump mechanism supplying the entire body with blood and one that amazes scientists to this day.

On average, your heart beats 100,000 times a day without you having to think about it. It doesn't take any time-outs; it doesn't go on vacation. It does its job every second of the day. The heart pumps 6,000 liters of blood through a network of vessels that cover 100,000 km throughout the body *every day*. In an average life span, the heart will beat over 2.5 billion times. The heart's valves consist of tissue so delicate that they are thinner than tissue paper, yet this is the strongest muscle in the human body.

It deserves repetition - the heart is a muscle. A muscle will wither away and *atrophy* or break down if not used regularly. When you go to bed, your heart rate goes down to conserve energy. All of this natural brilliance, and it only weighs between 9 and 11 ounces! The whole point of the heart is first to pump blood to the lungs to pick up oxygen, then pump that oxygen-rich blood throughout the body. It's that simple.

The Lungs

Twenty thousand breaths are taken every day without our conscious awareness. We breathe in and out to provide oxygen that totals over a thousand liters of air, or 340 liters of pure oxygen. Our lungs are a perfect example of coordination. The lungs are needed to provide oxygen to the cells. After being breathed in, oxygen passes to the heart through the blood. This process occurs by allowing the diaphragm to contract (move down), causing the lungs to expand as we inhale or inspire.

When you exhale, the muscles relax, and the air releases out of the lungs. When you inhale, the diaphragm and the intercostal muscles contract. This function allows the chest cavity to expand, which then causes the lungs to expand. A change in the pressure inside the lungs occurs, allowing air to enter the lungs. When you exhale, the diaphragm and intercostal muscles relax, causing the pressure inside the lungs to be greater than the pressure outside, which releases the air out of the body.

During this entire process of air exchange, the body absorbs the oxygen from the air through a series of blood vessels called pulmonary capillaries. These capillaries are tiny vessels located next to the *alveoli* of the lungs, the smallest functional element of the lung itself. The scale of this exchange is microscopic and is quite complicated.

Blood consists of three types of cells: red blood cells (which carry oxygen and carbon dioxide on a protein called *hemoglobin*), white blood cells (part of the immune system), and platelets (which assist in clotting). Initially, during inspiration (inhalation), the hemoglobin in the red blood cells has a carbon dioxide molecule attached to it, which must be released. As the red blood cell enters the alveoli, oxygen swaps place with the carbon dioxide molecule. Oxygen from the lung carries on towards the heart, while carbon dioxide remains in the lung. Upon expiration (exhalation), the carbon dioxide releases from the alveoli and out into the atmosphere.

Thus, the primary function of the lungs is to maintain high levels of oxygen within the blood and remove carbon dioxide from the blood. This fantastic process is carefully regulated through an elaborate system within the nervous system. Within this system, every aspect of the breathing process gets closely monitored. Oxygen needs to be bound, and carbon dioxide has to release. Remember, this process is taking place every second -- on average 20-30,000 times a day. It is something we do not need to control actively.

Skin

As the largest organ, the skin comprises 16% of our body weight. The skin serves many functions. It protects us from infections due to injury. It serves as a protective coating from the effects of harmful ultraviolet through the production of melanin. Exposure to the sun produces the pigment melanin. Vitamin D3, the precursor to Vitamin D, essential for forming healthy bones, is found in melanin.

The skin, though very thin, protects the body as well as excretes toxins from the body. Sweating is the body's way of eliminating toxins through the skin. There are three primary areas this happens - through the armpits, the groin area, and behind the knee. Toxins expel through the skin via the most superficial blood vessels.

This system also regulates the temperature inside the body, especially during hot and cold conditions. It does this through a staggering supply of blood that runs along the outermost layer of the skin. In hot climates, blood flow to the skin can be up to seven times higher than the norm, while superficial blood flow is almost undetectable during cold conditions. Through conduction, convection, and radiation, the heat transfer to the surface allows the body to cool.

The skin also acts as a protective border. It is, in a sense, part of the immune system, identifying and preventing foreign invaders from entering the body. Upon detection of an unwanted element, it then signals for the cavalry. It creates a cascade reaction from the immune system, thus stimulating the body's ability to protect itself from its environment.

Let us not forget that the skin also allows us to communicate with the world through its extraordinary sense of touch and feel. It also responds to sudden changes in our emotions and is the body's primary organ of sexual attraction.

The Liver

The liver is located along the lower right aspect of the abdomen. What is so important about the liver? The liver is like the body's Swiss army knife and has many functions, spanning most of our life processes. It connects to the gall bladder and is involved in the absorption of fats and fat-soluble vitamins.

The liver has a significant role in protecting the body from harmful substances as blood flows into the liver via the stomach and intestines. The liver stores and releases energy while it controls blood sugars. It can create sugar when required in a process called *glycogenolysis,* and it can store sugar for later in a process called *gluconeogenesis.*

The liver regulates fat storage, aids in digestion through bile production, and regulates blood clotting. It produces hormones in our bodies and filters blood. The liver's function is essential, especially if we are removing bacteria and toxins.

The liver also creates cholesterol, which is necessary for every cell in the body. It produces Vitamin D and stores minerals such as iron. Again, this is all done without your awareness. It doesn't take a break; the liver works all the time.

The Kidneys

Most of us are born with two kidneys. They are located bilaterally just below the rib cage. Each kidney has millions of tiny tubules called nephrons. These nephrons filter the blood that circulates through their structure.

The kidney reabsorbs crucial substances needed for the normal function of the body. The kidneys' primary role is to filter waste from the body and retain required substances, such as proteins, glucose, minerals, and water. As this is all done, the kidney can maintain *electrolyte* balance, which governs blood concentration and water usage in our system.

Kidneys are vital for the production of Vitamin D, which helps maintain healthy bones. They produce hormones that regulate blood pressure and stimulate the hormone *erythropoietin*, which is essential to make red blood cells.

The Eyes

The human eyeball is a sphere approximately four centimeters in size. Millions of cells allow for the remarkable feat of vision to take place. Scan the room and take a look at what you see. Try to absorb it all. The sense of sight is a miracle! The complicated physics of transforming light into the moving picture you see and register is incredible.

We can see about one million colors and their exponential array of shades. This is almost impossible to comprehend, especially when we tend to identify colors as simply red, blue, green, yellow, black, and white. This seeming superpower is part of a complex physical property called the Planck Distribution, named for the scientist Max Planck. This perceptual system allows different shades of color, light, and other shapes to be absorbed and understood almost instantly.

The Ears

Our hearing mechanism is a miraculous creation allowing us to hear the most beautiful songs, the most relaxing sounds of the ocean, and the voices of our loved ones. The ear's function involves the tiniest bones in the body, namely the middle ear's malleus, incus, and stapes.

To understand hearing better, follow the bouncing ball! The outer ear picks up vibrations from our environment, transmitting to the eardrum, creating patterns of movement for the middle ear bones. These movements amplify the vibration and relay the signal to a fluid in a structure called the *cochlea*. Once in the cochlea, highly sensitive cells receive the movement and finally pass the signal to the auditory nerve. This cranial nerve then plugs in directly to the brain for interpretation of the signal.

Muscles

There are 650 muscles within the human body. They propel us forward and allow us to maintain our balance in relation to gravity. They protect our internal organs, as well as provide a tremendous level of strength. If all the muscles in the human body were to pull in the same direction, they would haul an estimated twenty-five tons.

There are three types of muscle tissue: cardiac, smooth, and skeletal. Cardiac muscle is only found in the heart and is incredibly unique to that organ. It can receive electrical impulses created by the *sinoatrial node (SA node),* also known as the heart's pacemaker, regulating the heart's pumping function.

Smooth muscle is the muscle that controls all the body's systems that do not require our input. Put another way, smooth muscle controls all our *involuntary* actions, including squeezing our digestive tract to move along food and allowing our diaphragm to contract so we can breathe. If you don't think about it and it works anyway, that's the brain controlling the smooth muscle, so don't worry about it!

That leaves skeletal muscle, which makes up 60-90% of your body weight, depending on gender and age. These are all the muscles you must contract voluntarily – you must choose for it to work. Most movement falls in this category, including exercise, standing, walking, and sitting.

We may realize the magnitude of the work the muscles do when we need to exert extra strength. However, there are so many functions they perform that we take for granted. When was the last time you consciously thought about raising your arm to reach for something or scratch your head? Muscles attach to bones via *tendons,* and by contracting, they can move joints.

The Skeletal System

The skeletal system consists of 213 bones. Most of these bones protect our internal organs and provide resiliency against forces. They allow us to walk upright and are specialized for movement. When two bones come together, they form a joint. Most major muscles pull on these bones to achieve movement by moving the joints, most of the time in coordination with other muscle groups.

There are many functions for the skeletal system, but forming red blood cells in the bone marrow is quintessential. When you think of bones, you immediately think of the skeleton on display, long thin ribs, and knobby bumps at the ends of arms and legs. This function of the bone marrow, the soft central area of long bones, is absolutely critical to our life. Indeed that is why patients with severe issues like leukemia desperately search for bone marrow donors – it could save their life. Red blood cells play a critical role in providing cells with oxygen and removing carbon dioxide from the blood.

We have been talking in great detail about the utter importance that the skeletal system has on your overall well-being as it relates to chiropractic. The skeletal system undergoes tremendous changes through our entire lifespan and can alter its shape depending on the active biomechanical forces. It makes complete sense to maintain these systems.

The skeletal system performs complex movements every day, yet it can function for 80-100 years without a problem. You can do a great deal through nutrition and exercise that is necessary to maintain the skeletal system. Maintenance is vital to minimize any harmful spinal decay that can occur at any age if you fail to maintain the skeletal system properly.

Chapter 12

Conditions and Illnesses Managed with Chiropractic

When most people think of a chiropractor, they tend to think of a doctor who manages and treats neck and back pain. Some might have a bit of a broader understanding of the science of chiropractic and know that chiropractors handle most conditions associated with the musculoskeletal system and the nervous system. What many people don't yet know is that chiropractic deals with every system in the body. It can *potentially* help with any and *every* condition a person may have. Chiropractic is one of the most helpful healthcare professions in its involvement in preventing many illnesses and diseases.

Since the central nervous impacts every organ and cell within the body, it would make sense that any problems with the nervous system would lead to issues with the organ's function. These problems lead to illness and disease in the worst cases and a general feeling of malaise in the most uncomplicated cases. Reduction in the signal that passes from the brain to body or vice versa leads to dis-ease, the opposite of health and balance.

Chiropractic cares for the nervous system by caring for the spine. The spine is the main conduit for the nervous system and protects the spinal cord and each nerve. It can also act antagonistically to the nervous system when vertebrae, that allow for movement and flexibility, become misaligned and hinder the function of the nervous system. This is a condition in chiropractic called spinal restriction or subluxation.

A study conducted in Sweden by 87 different chiropractors sought to determine how patients responded to routine chiropractic care other than benefits directly related to the musculoskeletal system. The study followed patients for twenty consecutive visits they were attending for any reason. A total of 1,504 patients completed questionnaires explaining where they noticed improvements in their symptoms for other conditions after receiving chiropractic treatment. Here are the fascinating results:

No. of Patients	Positive Improvements in Non-Musculoskeletal Symptoms
98	Easier to breathe
92	Improved digestive function
49	Clearer/better/sharper vision
34	Improved circulation
10	Less ringing in the ears
8	Acne/eczema better
7	Dysmenorrhea better
6	Asthma/allergies better

There has not been extensive research on every condition that has improved with chiropractic care yet. Chiropractic research still has a long way to go to establish some strong correlations to conditions outside of back pain, neck pain, and headaches. Much of the trouble in getting relevant research together is the subjective nature of the adjustment. It relies on the experience of a practitioner to palpate, evaluate, and then diagnose. The technique that he or she uses, despite extensive training, cannot be *exactly* the same from adjustment to adjustment. Therein lies a source of error that reduces the quality of research.

The other major stumbling block for chiropractic research involves the cause and effect relationship. The mechanism for which, say, vision becomes sharper following a spinal adjustment is not well understood. Despite the participant experiencing the change, there is no established pathway to explain *how* that happened. Chiropractors hypothesize that pressure reduces on a neural pathway, but more technologically driven research is required to prove this beyond a reasonable doubt. Besides the obvious "I did X, and then Y happened" report, several reported non-mechanical improvements have still yet to be proven by in-depth research.

On an almost daily basis, in our very own offices, we experience some exciting changes, especially in non-musculoskeletal situations. A long-time patient always reports seeing colors more vividly after a cervical adjustment. Another patient says that they slept exceptionally well immediately after their session. One more patient experienced an improvement in his battles with erectile dysfunction. While the research may not indicate that chiropractic care can improve these issues, the patients themselves can bear witness to their resolution. The omnipresent medical disclaimer – *results may vary* – applies here, as a person's unique individual history may significantly impact the outcome experienced.

The following pages are details of other far-too-prevalent conditions worldwide that improve through proper diet, exercise, and routine chiropractic care.

High Blood Pressure

High blood pressure (BP), or hypertension, is a condition where the force of the blood against the arteries is too strong, thus making the heart have to work harder at pumping blood. The two numbers associated with a blood pressure reading are *systolic* (the top number) and *diastolic* pressure (the bottom number). If your blood pressure reads 120/80, your systolic pressure is 120, and your diastolic pressure is 80. Systole or systolic pressure refers to the force blood is pushed out of the heart. Diastole or diastolic pressure refers to pressure on the arteries as the heart relaxes between beats. Too much force in either direction over time can lead to an overworked heart. If this occurs, it can cause the heart to become enlarged and creates a dangerous platform for future heart disease.

Experts don't exactly know what causes hypertension, but the risk factors are apparent. The most significant risk factor is family history. Suppose your older family members tend toward high blood pressure. In that case, you are likely to develop the condition, even if you do everything else in your power to live a healthy lifestyle.

Temporary rises in blood pressure can occur by certain foods, caffeine, medications, and even stress. These short-term spikes are not as dangerous as the long-term effects. The key takeaway here is to manage diet and exercise, so that blood pressure spikes are not prolonged.

Medical doctors treat hypertension with a complete arsenal of medications. Some medications open up the blood vessels and allow for pressure-free passage. Others thin the blood, reducing its viscosity. Chances are, if you start medicines for high blood pressure, you will remain on them for life, and the recommendations from medical doctors usually align with that.

Diet and exercise, as with all aspects of good health, are your number one defenses in controlling high blood pressure. Chiropractors work with patients to ensure a healthy lifestyle and an adequate amount of exercise. We try to facilitate movement over all else, armed with knowledge on how beneficial exercise can be.

Misalignments in the spine can restrict nerve signals that regulate blood pressure. The top area of the thoracic spine is primarily responsible for the heart and coronary arteries. Also, the first cervical vertebra is associated with blood supply and blood pressure regulation. By getting regular preventative chiropractic adjustments, patients can optimize blood flow by removing restrictions in the upper-middle back and the neck.

An interesting chiropractic fact on blood pressure pertains specifically to India. Perhaps the most well-known person of Indian origin received Chiropractic care to help manage issues with high blood pressure. Indeed, historical reports indicate that Mahatma Gandhi was suffering from hypertension in 1942. And after being treated for three months by an American chiropractor, Dr. Peter Boike, his issues had improved drastically, and he was able to continue his freedom-fighting efforts.

The first step in managing your blood pressure is to get a complete family history and lifestyle history. If you are an overweight smoker, the first line of attack would be to quit smoking and lose some weight. Both of these controllable factors contribute to high blood pressure significantly. If this patient opted for chiropractic care, a complete examination would ensue, followed by a treatment plan for exercise and adjustments. Adjustments to the spine would help remove any restrictions discovered in the evaluation.

Over the years, I have had several patients visit the clinic with either pain in their neck or back. Upon checking their vitals, I noticed that their blood pressure was through the roof. Some patients were referred to emergency care at the nearest hospital since these cases could become profoundly serious very quickly. In such cases, the patient was often not even aware their blood pressure was so dangerously high! In other less severe circumstances, we have had a steady number of cases that show considerable reductions to BP following an adjustment. Again, the available scientific research does not conclude that chiropractic can consistently produce significant changes to blood pressure, but the examples in our clinic show otherwise.

High Cholesterol

Another condition impacted by family history is high cholesterol. Diet is the primary factor in lowering the bad cholesterol known as LDL, or low-density lipoprotein. Diet and exercise can also increase "good" cholesterol (HDL cholesterol) or high-density lipoprotein, which works as a cleansing agent to remove LDL cholesterol. If diet alone does not balance out the cholesterol issues in your bloodstream, a visit to the chiropractor can help.

Just as with hypertension, family history has much to do with cholesterol levels. The liver produces eighty percent of cholesterol made by the body. Even a low cholesterol diet can make lowering cholesterol difficult if you have a family history of high cholesterol. Again, chiropractic can ensure there is less interference between nerve signals and the liver. This way, the correct regulatory messages are sent to the liver, and it is more likely to produce the proper amount of cholesterol needed for cell development in the body. This theoretical link between chiropractic and improved cholesterol metabolism is not well understood but seems feasible given the connection between chiropractic and its role in optimizing the nervous system.

Since the liver is crucially involved with the filtration of the blood and all duties related to cholesterol processing, it would make sense that we leave the liver uninhibited or overloaded handling other materials. Consumption of alcoholic beverages is one of the main inhibitors of liver function. Abstaining from alcohol can give your liver a much-needed break from processing toxins and provide your cholesterol issues with some relief. Further, a liver cleanse could stimulate the function of the organ from the inside out. Discuss any types of cleanses or detoxifications with your health practitioners before starting, especially if other health issues are present.

The simplest liver detoxification that I advocate is simple on paper but much harder to follow. However, if you're able to handle it, you end up feeling more energized, refreshed, and you also can lose a bit of weight along the way. The cleanse involves three weeks of exceptionally clean eating, with strict adherence to some of the rules. Some rules must be maintained throughout the 3-week cleanse; some rules only apply to the first half, and another set of rules apply only to the second half. The mandatory rules to follow for the duration of the three weeks include:

- No caffeine

- No alcohol

- No tobacco

- No nuts

- No dairy

- No sugar

- 3L of water per day, minimum

- 1-2 scoops of carbohydrate-free whey protein per day (typically between 20-30g of protein per scoop)

Kind of hardcore. Nobody said it would be easy! The first half of the cleanse looks like this:

Days 1-10, strictly vegetarian

- o No meat, eggs, or fish

- o No limit on vegetable or fruit consumption, but aim for 2/3 of the vegetables to be eaten raw

- o 1 cup of brown rice (cooked) or 1 cup of lentils PER DAY

- o Avoid starchy vegetables like carrots, potatoes (can be eaten but in limited quantity)

The first two to three days for someone not used to eating like this is absolute torture. Coming from a coffee enthusiast like myself, the hardest thing for me to let go of was my morning cuppa. Withdrawal-like symptoms are common – headaches, fatigue, and irritability are all part of the process. Completely stopping all added sugars in your diet will elicit cravings, so be firm in your decision to take on this challenge. Even a taste of something sweet will start your process over again, extending the duration of your cleanse.

Days 11-21

- o Introduction of chicken, turkey, eggs, and fish (max 1-2 servings per day)

Additional supplements are allowed. My recommendations include psyllium fiber (isabgol), multivitamins, and omega-three fish oil. A word of caution – this cleanse is meant to introduce dietary changes and habits. Instantly reverting to the carbohydrate and fried food diets you just gave up will create a bit of chaos in your system.

Gradually add foods that you haven't eaten in 3 weeks, and make sure you eat them sparingly, as a treat only.

After this cleanse, not only will you lose some 'extra' weight your body was holding on to, your body will be able to process fats and cholesterol much better. I experience immense changes to my energy levels, mood, and even the quality of my sleep. I feel like my athletic activities improve, and I generally have a much sunnier outlook on life! I try to do this cleanse once or twice a year and have been doing it for almost ten years!

Diabetes

Diabetes is a condition in which the body either does not produce enough insulin or does not process it properly in converting sugar to energy. In a sense, the untreated diabetic would be starving himself to death even while eating plenty of food. Type II diabetes is especially apparent in India, where the number of diabetics is the highest in the world. Simply being of south Asian descent is enough to label you "at-risk" for diabetes.

People with diabetes get grouped into three different categories. Some are born with the condition and often have it recognized by the time they are toddlers or pre-school-aged (juvenile diabetes). The second type of genetically diabetic disease is Type I diabetes, where the immune system attacks the cells of the pancreas that produce insulin. Finally, there is type II diabetes, formerly referred to as adult-onset diabetes. Until about 20 years ago, only the very elderly became diabetic due to organs shutting down slowly with age. Another group of adults who suffered higher rates of diabetes were clinically obese.

Today, diabetes is running rampant and mostly because there is such a high percentage of the population that is obese. Obesity is defined as being more than 30% overweight. There are now over 135 million Indians with the condition, almost four times the entire population of Canada! The number of obese people in the US rose by one-third between 1990 and 1998, according to statistics by the American Diabetes Association (ADA). This trend exists around the world. This growing group includes children, where more and more children with type II diabetes are obese at ages as young as 6.

According to the ADA, diabetics have two to four times the risk of having a heart attack at a young age. The key to controlling type II diabetes is, you guessed it, exercise and maintaining a healthy weight. In other words, it's an entirely *reversible* condition that requires attention, planning, and dedication.

The pancreas is responsible for controlling the production and use of insulin. Restoring proper function to the pancreas is impossible once damaged, so preventative care in allowing the pancreas to function at its optimal level is where chiropractic care can help. Prevention is essential for "pre-diabetics," which accounts for approximately 80 million Indian nationals. Again, optimization of the pancreatic function is a deductive step in the pathway of chiropractic care. As the operation of the nervous system improves via chiropractic adjustments, it quite possibly can enhance the function of the pancreas.

Stress

Emotional stress affects men and women in different ways, and specifically, the types of stress on a woman's system will result in various conditions. Many people will get headaches, suffer from insomnia, or develop digestive problems when the stresses of daily life go unchecked.

One example is that stress releases hormones that impact women, specifically by creating an imbalance in their overall endocrine system. Since the nervous system is the system that can regulate and bring back equilibrium to all other systems, it makes sense to use chiropractic care to free up the nervous system to do its job.

Everyone can incorporate lifestyle changes into their routines. These not only include good eating habits and exercise but ways to reduce stress mentally. It has been my experience that when a patient is under tremendous pressure, it affects their ability to deal with pain effectively. More specifically, stress increases a patient's sensitivity to pain, which could cause them to rate their pain higher than it would in non-stressful times.

To illustrate this to my patients, I usually use a two-scenario example. In scenario A, imagine watching a light-hearted comedy in a dark room. You laugh a lot, and the movie has a happy ending. Once the movie ends, you turn off the TV and head to your room. In the process, you stub your little toe against the coffee table. In scenario B, you're watching a gripping, intense drama with a sad, emotional ending. Once again, you stub your toe in the dark against the coffee table. In which scenario, A or B, would you experience more pain?

If you chose scenario B, you'd be correct. The reason for this involves emotional stress and the lack of it in scenario A. The emotional angst caused by the disappointing end in scenario B's movie illustrates how stress can influence your perception of everyday aches and pains. Same coffee table, same poor stubbed pinky toe. Different pain experienced! People who are under the gun, who are constantly being bombarded with life's challenges, or are fighting battles on multiple fronts are prone to experiencing more pain. And as we discussed in other chapters, stress that is prolonged and not dealt with adequately festers, ultimately becoming much worse than if it resolved early on.

I have found that Chiropractic care does wonders for stress. Whether it is the hands-on approach to healthcare, the therapeutic touch as it were, or the ability for chiropractors to listen to and empathize with their patients, we regularly see patients describe their stress levels as reduced post-session.

When chiropractic is not enough to break through the stress clouds, we are alert enough to recommend mental health professionals. We always recommend mental health counseling for patients who are having a more challenging time with handling stress. Counseling is a non-invasive, non-allopathic method of restoring normal, healthy thought processes and can help organize confusing thoughts and complicated ideas.

Especially in India, the view of mental health counseling is almost taboo, where patients fear being labeled as 'crazy.' Just as we would seek care for an aching muscle or joint, our brains also need help. Talking to your doctor about counseling is a great start. Many of us have situations where we have taken on too much commitment or are just unaware of what to do next. Counseling is a gentle way of sorting out your feelings and allowing you to arrive at conclusions that are best suited for you.

Counseling offers the help of a *neutral* third party. If we discuss an issue we're having with someone, the chances are that person is close to you somehow - a friend, family member, or co-worker perhaps. These people typically want you to be happy and try to help by offering words of support and encouragement. They may suggest solutions for you or join in your misery, adding fuel to the fire. Unfortunately, these people are biased towards you, may benefit from you temporarily avoiding your issues, and may not always offer you solutions that could help improve the source of your confusion, or worse, may confuse you further! A counselor is neutral in that they have no vested, *emotional* interest in your outcome. This fact allows their input to be unbiased, objective, and superior to your close friend's. They are there to support you, listen to you, and help you organize your mind.

Alzheimer's and Dementia

Alzheimer's disease is sexist! For unknown reasons, it affects many more women than men. There are approximately 4 million Indians with Alzheimer's, and about half of the population over 85 has the disease. There are also no known causes or cures for this disease that leaves victims with severe memory loss – even to the point that they cannot remember to eat or recognize loved ones. The only recent discoveries have included identifying an enzyme in the brain that builds up as a plaque and may trigger the disease.

There are some effective treatments for the symptoms of early dementia. The most hopeful evidence comes from studies where the herb Ginkgo Biloba is used to repair and regenerate the tiniest capillaries in the brain, releasing the blood needed to nourish the brain. Chiropractic care also removes the restriction to nerves that communicate with and nourish brain cells.

It is essential to differentiate between dementia that occurs more often as people age – sometimes referred to as a "senior moment" when we forget what we were going to say or the name of a good friend – and full-blown, diagnosed Alzheimer's. There are periods of less mental clarity that can occur with age but do not have to be an inevitable part of the aging process.

Although I cannot say with any amount of certainty that Chiropractic care can improve the conditions of Alzheimer's or dementia, I can say that at least with two specific patients, we did see improvement in their conditions throughout their treatment. In one of these cases, the patient would completely forget that he was in pain, only to be in agony moments later. This ebb and flow of extreme pain and relative calm was putting enormous strain on his family members. With short, gentle procedures, we were able to restore this gentleman's daily function to a point where he could walk, speak, and even request a visit to the office! His improvement was so noticeable that his neighbors in his apartment were all curious about how he could get well so suddenly (it also resulted in several new patients!).

Fibromyalgia Syndrome (FMS)

Fibromyalgia Syndrome (FMS), or just fibromyalgia (FM), is a relatively unusual condition, and for the record, we're only discussing it here because of its prevalence in India. Experts estimate that about 10 million people suffer from this disorder in India; however, I cannot justify using it as a diagnosis based on the weak research for this condition. However, for those it affects, it is an all-consuming way of life compounded by medical mismanagement. FMS restricts people's everyday life activities due to tenderness in the joints and muscles that the condition ultimately controls them.

FMS is a chronic condition marked by tenderness and pain in many different points throughout the body. Through extensive and non-conclusive research, the root of the problem is either neurochemical, peripheral, or soft-tissue related. There are also hormonal imbalances found in patients with FMS that seem to correlate. The nervous system and endocrine system, which encompass all of the hormones, are closely interconnected. In chiropractic, we view and understand that all systems connect to the nervous system, so it is understandable that chiropractic can help those with FMS.

And that's where I'll interrupt this train of thought to bring you my unadulterated opinion of this issue. Fibromyalgia was diagnosed with the clinician pressing on a patient's body to determine whether pain was present. If 10 out of 18 points were tender, this patient was diagnosed with FM. While that practice has now been replaced with thorough history taking, it still seems that the research community is out to lunch. Far too many patients have claimed to be diagnosed with this label.

Unfortunate patients get surprisingly unclear diagnoses by prominent physicians because "it can't be anything else." This, my good friends, is what I would unceremoniously call a "garbage can diagnosis." I can imagine the thought process of the frustrated physician going through the case history. "It hurts everywhere? All the time? And there were no accidents? You just woke up, and everything hurt? Does nothing help? Hmmm…" "We don't know what to call it, so we'll just slap this label on it, let's call it Fibromyalgia."

Experts have zeroed in on some potential neurological causes for FM. But there seems to be no auto-immune activity (where the body attacks its own cells), no issue with inflammation, and no specific damage to muscles or joints. A telling statement from rheumatology.org, the leading resource for all autoimmune conditions, suggests that there is still no clear understanding of what FM is - or if it's anything at all. Genes alone do not cause FM. No blood tests or medical imaging can detect FM. Under criteria needed for diagnosis of FM, the website lists "no other health problem that would explain the pain and other symptoms" – in a nutshell – the very definition of "garbage can diagnosis."

An exceedingly high number of cases show the presence of trauma, whether psychological or physical, as a 'trigger' for the pain. In one case I've worked on, a patient got stuck in an elevator. Upon emerging from the elevator, she immediately felt piercing pain all through her body. When she came to see me, she had already dealt with the pain for more than four years. With regular discussion, adjusting, and exercises, she found that her pains mysteriously vanished. She was able to sleep better, her appetite returned, and her ability to play golf on weekends improved. Her therapist emailed me and confirmed my suspicions. Her counseling sessions were progressing, and her mood was noticeably better.

When there was an unfortunate demise in her family, and she could not attend her visits for two weeks, she returned with the entire situation reversed. Her stress, emotional fragility, and unresolved mental trauma played a significant role in her pain. Upon increasing her counseling sessions and falling back into a routine of exercise and adjustments, her condition once again improved. Her attempts at maintaining consistency over the years were minimal, her husband later confided. For the first time in four years, she felt well enough to hit a golf ball off the tee, only because I convinced her that she needed consistency and routine.

The hardest thing about patients being diagnosed with "FMS" (I will henceforth use quotations to indicate my feelings about the "syndrome") is that it plays poorly to an already compromised psyche. It serves as a label, and to a degree, it can be relieving for the mind, as in "I have *something* with a name." The patient believes that it's no longer a phantom problem affecting the whole body, it has a name, and they can share it with family and friends.

In some patients, the diagnosis serves as a shield. "I would do that, but I can't because of my fibro," is something an actual patient has said to me. The patient became so entangled in her arbitrary diagnosis that it started to become her identity. She had even told me that she was 'the sick friend' in her friend circle. In others, it's a source of constant attention, where family and well-wishers lavish their efforts to make life easier.

My clinical mind empathizes with patients in these chronic pain conditions. It's painful, and it's *tiring* to be in pain constantly. Chronic pain, chronic fatigue, insomnia, they're all connected, as in a vicious cycle. If you increase one, you have no choice but to increase the others. But intervene on one, and now you have a window of opportunity. Exercise, a magic pill for loads of mental health issues, can work here once the inertia of moving the body wears off.

Although I doubt the so-called syndrome, I will continue this discussion out of respect for patients going through these exact things. I apologize for the digression. As we were…

Chiropractic has been highly effective in helping those who suffer from "FMS." The relief from pain patients with "FMS" receive is from the adjustments and procedures that get the nerves, joints, and muscles into optimal working order. Because those with FMS also suffer tenderness in all the nodules in their muscles, chiropractic care can help decrease the sensitivity to pain by assisting the body to metabolize waste and eliminate toxins properly.

There are lifestyle changes that go hand in hand with chiropractic to help relieve the pain of "FMS." Dietary changes that include adequate amounts of magnesium help the patient to maintain proper pH balance. Better pH levels allow better nerve transmission to the other nerves and muscles. Ideal hydration and adopting an anti-inflammatory diet have also shown promise in keeping pain levels down.

Keeping a routine schedule that includes plenty of exercise and sleep also helps alleviate "FMS" symptoms. Exercise, 20-30 minutes per day, done in the late afternoon or evening, is most effective and promotes sound sleep -- another way to battle "FMS" symptoms. Doing exercises in a swimming pool is great because it places less pressure or weight on sensitive muscles due to buoyancy.

Chemical Addiction

Chemical addiction can be a lifelong battle for those who struggle with drug dependency -- prescription or recreational. However, new studies by the American College of Addictionology and Compulsive Disorders (ACAD) in Miami, Florida, evaluate the role of chiropractic in treating addicts. This preliminary research is gaining traction and sheds light on another avenue of chiropractic care.

A triple-blind study conducted in conjunction with the Florida Chiropractic Society found that a person receiving chiropractic care has a 97 percent retention rate of staying off of addictive drugs. This incredible result is ten times the rate of all people who complete a drug rehabilitation program. The ACAD specifically approached the chiropractic community because of its drug-free approach to health care.

With any drug rehabilitation program, retention is the key. Many people can enter and stay clean for the brief time they are in rehab, only to relapse once they return to their everyday lives and routines. This chiropractic study on addicts focused on removing restrictions in the spine that got in the way of the normal functioning of the nervous system and specifically the signals that deal with dependency and additive responses.

The most challenging part of overcoming an addiction can be the physical responses of withdrawal once the drug is no longer in the body. As with sugar that we discussed earlier, craving drives the addict to seek out the drug repeatedly – and at just about any cost. The drug-free approach taken by chiropractic can eliminate the physical symptoms of withdrawal. Once that urge is no longer a driving force, the addict can better deal with the more emotional reasons they may have sought the drug.

Chiropractic has taken strides in the treatment of people with chemical dependencies. Life Chiropractic College in Marietta, Georgia, has the first chiropractic program to address treatments for chemical dependency specifically. Medical schools may have courses directed toward educating the doctor about what drugs can treat the addiction to other drugs. Still, it is at Life Chiropractic College that a full-blown program dedicated to this initiative exists.

Chapter 13

The Nervous System – Central to Good Health

Upon conception, the first feature that developed in all of us was the brain. Next, our body produces a protective case, a bony layer called the cranium. Following the cerebrum (the 'main part' of the brain), the spinal cord develops, a long nerve-like projection directly descending from the brain. That, too, became encased in a protective armor called the vertebrae or spinal column.

The next part to be developed in-utero was the spinal nerve roots, which are extensions of the spinal cord. Ultimately, those spinal nerve roots create spinal nerves, which become surrounded by embryonic tissue. The brain receives stimulation from the embryonic tissue via feedback from the nervous system. Only after all this development has occurred the other systems in the body develop.

This very brief embryology lesson illustrates how crucial the nervous system is to sustaining life. Indeed, the nervous system is what controls all the systems in the body. If you were to look up "nervous system" in Webster's Dictionary, you would find it defined as the following: "The master control system of the body that controls all other systems of the body."

The nervous system consists of three different areas. The first is the brain. It is the originator of the messages that require distribution to all the cells, tissues, organs, and systems of the body. The second part of the nervous system is the spinal cord. Think of it as the superhighway of the nervous system. It is a complex system that has routes to every corner of our body. The third part of the nervous system is the spinal nerve. Think of this as an exit off the main highway. Without these exits, you can never really get to a specific destination. From these spinal nerves, peripheral nerves branch off exponentially, creating a vast system of nerves and nerve endings, allowing us to feel, understand, and sense the environment around us and respond to changes.

The brain weighs only three pounds. Despite only needing the energy of a ten-watt bulb, the functions of the brain are truly staggering. Some say that the brain is so functionally complete and complex that you would need two buildings the size of the Empire State Building with today's technology that could rival its power. As farfetched as that may seem, despite the inroads today's technology is making, the brain is unique.

Let me explain further. The brain can perform billions of operations simultaneously. Billions! A computer can only perform a few tasks at a time. A computer can perform the task at astounding speeds, but it can only execute them a few at a time. Therefore, for the computer to replicate the total capacity of the nervous system, you would need a massive system enabling the computer to perform complex tasks, billions of them at the same time. Not to be outdone, the brain can send and receive signals at over 400 km/h. In situations involving life and death, we want that ability to send and receive messages as fast as possible!

Here is another way to emphasize the importance of the nervous system. If you cut the nerve to the lungs, how would the lung know what to do? Think of the lung as an appliance, and the spinal cord is the circuit. If the circuit breaker isn't allowing energy to flow into the outlet that supplies the device, the device is not going to work. It's the same with the cells, tissues, organs, and systems of the body.

The Workings of the Nervous System

Every cell in the body has an intelligent design. The cells which make up the tissues and the tissues that make up the organs also have this ingenuity. In the healthy organs chapter, we outlined some of the remarkable processes the body can perform, again, by intelligent design. The complicated systems perform many tasks every second without us having to provide input. If there is damage in the body, the body is equipped with mechanisms to fight against it and protect from further harm. This troubleshooting failsafe is all orchestrated by the nervous system.

Let's delve back into philosophy for a moment. Some say that there is internal "divine" guidance that steers all the functions of the body. It knows what substance to produce at the exact time needed. The number of neuronal connections within our body is astounding. There are more possible connections in the brain than there are combinations of phone numbers within India. Just imagine that number!

So what prevents our body from performing its best? What prevents this splendid orchestra from playing its tune called health?

Interference with the nervous system can have serious complications. Think about this for a moment. If I'm on the phone and I'm giving you very detailed instructions on how to get from point A to point B, and all of a sudden your phone begins to break up, will you be able to accurately receive the directions you need to get to your destination? This little goof-up is not because you are incompetent; there was a digital disruption in our communication. The signal did not get passed efficiently.

The key is to maintain as close to 100% communication within every aspect of the body. Admittedly, this is a tall task. Researchers are still learning about the mechanisms within our bodies that communicate crucial messages. Historically, these messages have not been interpreted fully. One example is fever. At first, fever was something that needed to stop as soon as possible. We now know that its purpose is to thwart foreign invaders like bacteria and viruses. By making the body unlivable (too hot) for these invaders, the fever actually *helps* you heal. Stopping the fever too soon with antipyretic drugs, for example, allows the bug to linger around, possibly delaying your infection from healing.

There are many examples of this type of conclusion that scrambles messages emotionally, physically, and nutritionally. Misunderstandings take place all the time. That is why I'm writing this book -- to give you a basic understanding of your body and what you can do immediately to reduce some of the confusion. This clarity should take your health to the next level. You have a very sophisticated body that needs a better understanding of how to provide it with the essential care it needs. Consider this book a user's manual for the body you've always known but never cared for optimally.

Suppose the entire nervous system is fully functioning and fully interactive, with all the cells, tissues, organs, and other systems in the body. In that case, the body can effectively and efficiently respond to dangerous conditions in the body. However, if the nervous system is not functioning correctly, it will create an imbalance or lack of ease (dis-ease).

The mindset that we have in regards to our bodies must be changed. Are we just to get by in a cruel world and play the cards we were dealt? Or is life a miracle, and are the bodies that we inhabit the temple of our souls? Do we have reverence for our bodies? Again, this book is a wake-up call for you. Realize that there is so much in all of us to stimulate health -- so much potential. Unfortunately, most of the time, through ignorance or apathy, the body just wastes away.

In the upcoming chapters, you will realize that our internal workings can be the most beautiful source of immuno-stimulation. Yet, it can also be the major source of disease creation. Dr. Gary Null, one of the leading health and fitness voices in the US, has stated that health breaks down into 25% nutrition, 25% exercise, and a whopping 50% mental attitude. If we have certain expectations and believe in them with conviction, those expectations can manifest in the physical world. In other words, you truly become what you think about, good or bad. What we must remember is that the intelligent design that created us at conception still flows through every cell in our body today, and we must honor that miracle.

I tell my patients that the body is providing us with signals, and we cannot ignore those signals. Again, I will stress one thing; I or any other chiropractor do not cure anything or anyone! The body does the curing. Despite not using medications and drugs or other invasive methods, how are chiropractors able to do so much good?

In a nutshell, chiropractors can stimulate the nervous system to function more effectively, whether by adjusting, prescribing exercise, or correcting lifestyle issues. The nervous system does the rest, guiding your body to perform better and more efficiently. The body receives pain signals at times, a flare to direct its attention towards an ongoing issue. Individually we may not have the capacity and understanding of what is happening, which is why we rely on the expertise of doctors.

The way I see it, you have two choices: use your body well, or abuse it. If you choose to abuse, you will suffer the consequences of natural processes. You get what you give, so to speak. So, if we are to attain incredible levels of health, we must first start with an equivalent level of gratitude and respect for our bodies. Please don't take it for granted.

When you realize that you have a choice to carve out of life what you want, to create a magical life full of passion, vibrancy, and possibility, then you must be grateful for what you have. Think about it. There are so many things for which you can and should be grateful. The practice of gratitude is also an ancient technique in meditation and has been used to treat everything from chronic pain and depression to headaches!

The body that you are in right now is doing everything it can to support you at this very moment. It is there to serve you. So, today, I want you to decide that you will no longer look at your body as something that 'deserves' a candy bar or a soda from now on. Think of it as one of the finest, exotic cars in the world, one that deserves and should receive only the best fuel, maintenance, and care.

If you owned a $100,000 racehorse, you would train it constantly. You would feed it the best food possible. Why? Because you spent all that money and you expect to get a return on your investment. Well, what do you suppose you and your health are worth? If you desperately needed one, how much would you be willing to pay for a liver transplant? How much for a kidney transplant? What's your heart worth? What's the price for your hearing? What would you trade for your vision? Can you now see how valuable and priceless you are? These questions are an exaggeration of a simple truth – we cannot put a price on health.

Philosophically, realize that you are here for a reason. You are here not to be a wandering generality but to be a meaningful specific; a person destined to achieve something worthwhile. You can't attain your heart's desires without the spark of energy derived from a true level of health and well-being. Begin today with a new appreciation that your life demands authentic, sustained energy, not just bouts of it. It deserves an upgraded level of health that rivals the idea you once thought of as acceptable.

Chapter 14

"Perfect" Posture

We've practiced this ever since we were toddlers (and probably even got punished for it!). In military and exercise programs, this is essential. Yet, most of us still struggle to keep it right. What is it? Our posture.

Let us start this discussion by saying there is no such thing as PERFECT POSTURE. It is a scale of only better and worse. Having poor posture leads to all sorts of problems for our bodies. Appearance-wise, poor posture makes our shoulders sag, round forward, and can result in a 'hunchback.' We can also have the appearance of someone feeling down or sad.

We tend to focus too much on the superficial signs of poor posture without realizing what insidious problems lay lurking ahead. One of the most significant risks of poor posture is the damage to your spine – the protective cover to our spinal cord, which holds us upright. Poor posture can also be debilitating to our muscles.

So, what makes the ideal posture? Athletic performance expert, Dax Moy, affirms that bad posture is one of the critical factors contributing to bad health in most developed countries. He explains that when the human frame is out of proportion, it results in poor posture. This eventually imposes a load on the body's vital organs and systems.

What Is Posture?

Before we talk about better posture, let's explain what posture is in the first place. If we get back to the basics, posture, at its core, is the way we bear our physique unconsciously (without thinking about it or controlling it). Our posture links with the way our brain reacts to its surroundings. It also interacts with the force of gravity exerted upon the body.

Physical Therapist Frank D'Ambrosio states that an ideal posture means that no area of your body bears unequal pressure when standing or sitting. Every time we stand, walk, sit, kneel, or bend, we are essentially pitting ourselves against gravity. In turn, gravity (a natural force) places strain on our muscles, ligaments, and joints. Good posture is equal to good balance.

D'Ambrosio has a perfect definition of good posture. He states that an architect uses the same laws of gravity when he drafts a new house or building design. And similar to a home or building with a bad foundation, a human body with poor posture is weaker and less tolerant of the stress we tend to go through later in our lives.

Dax Moy further elaborates that poor posture is the leading culprit behind arthritis, back strain, fatigue, and headaches. As you can see, left unresolved, the problems and risks that arise are numerous when you have poor posture.

One of the most common reasons people visit my practice is for the treatment of headaches. I recall a banking professional, who had terrible migraines, at least 3-4 times per week, who came to our clinic after trying many different procedures. After performing a physical check-up on her, we found lots of misalignment in her cervical spine that restricted her range of motion. More obviously, her head was quite a bit forward in comparison to her shoulders. Our postural screen revealed much the same. According to our posture analysis software, the weight of her head, which should have been around the 10lb mark, actually weighed 22lbs based on the amount of pressure it was exerting on her cervical spine!

Following a treatment lasting six weeks, the headache frequency of the patient decreased to only one headache per month, and her posture visibly improved. There was still room for improvement, but she had shown a substantial transformation in her posture and headache frequency- she no longer resorted to painkillers to ease her headaches. She understood that her problems didn't develop overnight, and she had the patience to allow some time for the treatment to work.

Body pain isn't the only effect of poor posture. It can also affect your mood. Here is an example - picture someone that is depressed or anxious and imagine how their stance appears. Do their shoulders point straight ahead? Is their head upright and alert? Or do they look somewhat sunken and withdrawn? This is an important finding, both biomechanically and psychologically. Scientists hypothesized that since the body physically responded to mood, perhaps the opposite was possible. In many studies over the years, researchers have found that indeed posture can also influence mood. For example, people who rated their mood as low (4 or below, on a 10 point scale) reported significant changes after actively improving their posture for 10-30 minutes. Measuring brain waves and serotonin levels (the brain's feel-good hormone) confirmed this outstanding result.

Why does this happen? Our brains have physical memory space for most of our bodily movements and emotional reactions to certain situations. Our feelings and emotions live in a part of our brain called "the limbic system" (or the emotional brain) found in the cerebrum. Dr. R. Joseph, in his report "Catatonia," studied patients with several minor wounds in their cerebrum. He explains that these people are in a catatonic state and suffer from apathy (partial or complete lack of feelings) and slow responses to external stimuli.

The standard transmission of signal would result in the limbic system relaying information to the frontal neocortex, a section of the brain that converts thought to movement. Dr. Joseph adds that lesions in the limbic system disengage the fibers needed to relay that signal, resulting in less movement and reaction to emotional stimuli. His studies concluded that the signaling between these two crucial parts of the brain was a two-way street, and that change in expression on one end would affect the other end.

The Connection Between Posture And Breathing

Based on recent research findings, poor posture can be incredibly destructive to healthy and essential breathing patterns. You don't need a scientist or doctor to make this connection; you can try it directly yourself. Try breathing while hunched forward. Now try it while maintaining a nice, tall spine. Which was easier? The key lies in the pressure exerted on our diaphragm.

When we mentioned breathing previously in this book, we saw that the diaphragm is responsible for expanding our lungs to receive the largest amount of air and oxygen from the atmosphere into our systems. When the diaphragm contracts (moves down), it allows the lungs and the chest cavity to enlarge so that air rushes in. When the diaphragm relaxes, the lungs and the chest relax too and push air out.

A gentle reminder - we breathe on average 20 - 30,000 times a day! If your diaphragm is blocked (because of bad posture), you won't be able to breathe in very deeply. This results in your cells getting less oxygen. As we mentioned earlier, cells that don't get enough oxygen cannot function at their best, leading to damage and disease. Great posture translates to a great functioning diaphragm and ultimately better function of the body's cells.

The Connection Between Posture And Headaches

Several studies demonstrate a clear link between poor posture and headaches and neck issues. The Cervical Spine Research Society in the US considers most headaches (70-80%) to be cervicogenic in nature. In more simple words, these headaches relate to the head, scalp, and neck and a particular nerve called the "trigeminal nerve." The issue is that headaches can stem from trauma (from a car crash or accidental fall), neurological problems, or even something as simple as dehydration.

In normal posture, the spine supports the head like a steel girder. However, when the head (which has an average weight of 10-12 pounds) is tilted forward in poor postural positions, it increases the pressure exerted on the spine. The resulting stress on the vertebrae, ligaments, and muscles leads to muscle spasms and accelerates degenerative changes. This stress will interfere with average blood circulation through the spinal muscles and affect the spine's overall function if this goes on for an extended period. Muscle spasm or muscle tension over long periods can also diminish the function of the muscle and create scar tissue, which is a less functional area within a muscle.

When it comes to tackling scar tissue in these situations, doctors aim to manipulate the tissue without any pain or tension. They commonly use IASTM (instrument-assisted soft tissue manipulation) or Graston, which can locate and treat scar tissue. This technique is one of the non-invasive tools used in treating chronic and painful problems resulting from damaged tissue. Another treatment option is cold laser therapy (also known as low laser therapy) which can also help decrease scar tissue.

Determining Good Posture

There are many opinions on what makes good posture. So how do you know what *good* posture is? There is one thing that most doctors, chiropractors, and physical therapists are unanimous about - we should balance our bodies from front to back, right to left, in as close to perfect symmetry as possible. The amount of weight and strain placed on our necks should be equally distributed.

From a chiropractic point of view, the natural spinal curves are a symbol of health. We have three such curves: lordosis in the cervical spine, kyphosis in the thoracic spine, and lordosis in the lumbar spine. Again, lordosis refers to a convex curve towards the front of the body (curve faces forward), and a kyphosis refers to a concave curve towards the front of the body (curve faces backward). With poor posture, these curves are often affected, creating degenerative changes along the way, and straightening the spine as a result. Restoration of the spinal curves is one of the main focuses of chiropractic care. One branch of chiropractic science, "chiropractic biophysics (CBP)," scientifically deduces the rate of curvature change for patients under treatment.

Despite such advances in science, there are situations where a chiropractor can't fully re-align the patient back to its original condition. The level of scarring of the ligaments along the spinal column greatly determines the prognosis of the patient. Additionally, other factors like age and lifestyle habits can influence the outcome.

Checking For Ideal Posture

As specified earlier, the ideal situation is perfect alignment and symmetry, both when viewing the spine from left to right and front to back. Looking in a mirror, beginning with your head, check for any type of rotation or sideways bending towards your right or left. Then check your hips to see if they are roughly at the same height. Next, check the position of your feet at rest. Are they slightly rotated inwards (pigeon-toed) or outwards (duck feet)? If you noticed any variation in these areas, you might have increased stress levels on the skeletal system and spine.

Dax Moy also suggests the following tips to improve posture. Ensure you consult your chiropractor first before trying these out to make sure they don't affect your treatment.

- Increase your range of motion through various exercises that enhance flexibility and stretch the tightened muscle groups.

- Perform balance exercises to assist your joints in adjusting to different movements. Pilates, Yoga, Alexander Technique, Tai Chi, and similar exercise programs are suitable for this purpose.

- Perform strengthening exercises in your daily exercise schedule. Preferably engage the postural muscles in your back.

- Adopt functional exercises into your workouts. Exercises and movements used in daily activities are most beneficial, no need to use machines.

Good posture is a game of balance – a few minutes of good posture won't matter if you are not paying attention to your posture the rest of the day. Consistency is king! Aim to get better every day.

Chapter 15

Exercise, Posture & Ergonomics

Exercise is crucial to good cardiovascular health and muscle tone, but it is also significant to posture. When muscle tone in the back is healthy, we naturally have better posture and can keep ourselves upright without too much thought. The back muscles help hold the spine erect (they're literally called *spinal erectors!*). With good posture, our shoulders are relaxed and not hiked up around our ears. Stress is a detractor for good posture. So, when we free ourselves from stress through meditation and exercise, we can see visible changes in our bodies. In a nutshell, good posture combines maintaining good muscle tone, reducing stress, and feeling comfortable overall.

The Effect on Muscle Strength & Bone Density

Are you worried about the hunch starting to form in your upper back? No, you don't have an abnormality like Quasimodo, although it is liable to get worse if you don't do something about it! In the short term, the spine won't permanently mold itself into a slouched position, but the muscle tone can become so weak that it cannot hold the spine up. However, poor posture can create bony wear and tear over a long time, some of which is irreversible.

A great deal of research has gone into the skeletal and muscular effects of exercise. In a conference on osteoporosis (low bone density) prevention, Dr. Robert A. Marcus reported the impact of exercise on muscle tone and bone density and how that affects overall health. The research revealed that Bone Mineral Density (BMD) didn't necessarily increase with moderate exercise, but without it, it most assuredly decreased. Only high-impact activities, such as jumping and running, showed an increase in BMD. However, even low-intensity, low-movement activities like standing helped maintain current levels of BMD.

The good news is, even without increasing BMD, muscle strength can improve with exercise. Building and maintaining muscle is especially imperative for the elderly, who cannot engage in many high-intensity activities that promote increases in BMD. Just by toning muscles, especially leg muscles, even those in their 90s can reduce the risk of serious injury if they fall.

The only group of people in the research conducted on BMD that had differing results was children. The time when a person is usually most active is childhood. Children can build a reserve of BMD that provides benefits throughout life. An inactive child might have problems with BMD as an adult. For any adult, however, to maintain adequate BMD, they must continuously exercise throughout their life.

Developing the back and improving posture include strengthening many other muscle groups. Some of these are:

- Abdominals

- Hamstrings

- Quadriceps

- Gluteus

- Front Neck

- Scapula (shoulder blade) supporting muscles

There are many practical exercises for each muscle group, all of which can fit any fitness level. Any activity that flexes the muscle and stretches it gently is generally considered good. For general health, it is better to do shorter repetitive sets than to exhaust the muscle completely when performing an exercise. Doing 10 or 12 repetitions is good for each group to start. Then you can gradually increase the number as the muscles become conditioned.

Depending on your needs, it is generally not necessary to overwork the muscles. It will lead to soreness, at the very least, and even more severe injury if not monitored carefully. If, for example, you were to lift weights using one muscle group, you would want to rest those muscles for a day before repeating those exercises. This strategy is especially true as you get into heavier weights for resistance.

Pilates

There are different types of exercises, some as old as 5000 years, that provide good strength to muscles. Pilates is a back-friendly method of toning that focuses on all of the large muscle groups. It not only strengthens muscles but increases flexibility gently and effectively. It is an easy program to adopt, irrespective of what fitness level you start.

Joseph Pilates developed the exercise program as a way to strengthen his own body. He was a sickly child and unable to do many everyday childhood activities others enjoyed. During World War I, he further tested his strengthening concepts as a nurse and used his exercises to increase mobility in disabled veterans.

Today, over 500 different Pilates exercises focus on strengthening the core muscles, centering, and breathing. Together, with concentration, those who implement Pilates exercises will quickly see improved posture and flexibility, along with the ability to balance in positions related to holding their center of gravity.

Ergonomics

Ergonomics is a science that studies how the human body responds to the forces of nature through physical activity. In Greek, the terms *ergon* (work) and *nomoi* (natural laws) combine to create the English word ergonomics.

The goal of ergonomics is to reduce injuries by being aware of how the everyday activities in which we engage affect our joints and muscles. There are three basic rules to ergonomics that, if applied, would significantly reduce muscle tension or repetitive stress injuries (RSI) common in the workplace. They include: changing body positions often, using the largest muscle group for any work that exerts force, and only working joints to the mid-point of their range of motion.

When speaking of ergonomics, it is essential to understand that there is *static work* and *force*. Static work refers to those tasks that require you to maintain the same position or use small movements for extended periods. This may include typing, standing at a lab bench while bending over a microscope, or sitting in a truck with one hand on the steering wheel day after day.

Force, as it relates to ergonomics, is all about how much the muscles have to work. If you use the wrong muscles for the job, there can be an injury. This tenet is not limited to lifting heavy objects but can even include flexing the neck muscles to bend the head forward or backward from an upright position. The action of bending forward alone adds four times the force on the lower neck vertebrae. So, if you have a job where your head is bent down looking over paperwork, you are putting excessive pressure on your neck.

The way to counteract the impact of static work and force on the muscles and bones is to become conscious of each movement and change positions frequently throughout the day. Again, remember to use the largest appropriate muscles for any task, as this minimizes the risk of injury. For example, while lifting a heavy object, use your powerful legs to push the object up, and not your poor aching back.

Ergonomics takes thought. Thinking about your posture and the different positions you assume in any given task is not something we naturally do. We simply try to be comfortable and will revert to less healthy positions to achieve comfort. The only time we give thought to our body's position or posture is when we are uncomfortable. We then seek to change to a more relaxed way of sitting, standing, or lying down, relieving any discomfort in the process. Again, there is not much thought to the process; we just move until it feels good.

Since we naturally put little thought into ergonomics, doctors and scientists have been doing the heavy lifting for us. They have created tools and methods to ease the stresses we put on our joints and muscles. One of the most notable ergonomic inventions of the 20th century includes the foam strip at the base of computer keyboards, which raises the wrists to a better position for the wrist joints. This piece of genius reduced the cases of carpal tunnel syndrome experienced by typists who often spend several hours each day in that position.

Likewise, office chairs with lumbar support encouraged better posture for desk dwellers. We also saw an increase in the use of headsets for receptionists who, before that, would often cradle the telephone receiver between their ear and shoulder while taking notes. In many offices, you will see the semi-seated workstation. This is a type of chair where you are neither sitting nor standing. It keeps the lower back aligned with the rest of the back and promotes good posture. That, in turn, relieves pressure on the spine and alleviates back pain, especially in the lower back.

Ergonomics goes even further into our everyday lifestyle than for office workers or others who engage in repetitive movement for most of their day. Simple changes in how we carry out daily activities can make a difference in how well our backs and joints are protected. Each applies the three basic principles of ergonomics stated earlier: adopting differing positions, using the largest muscles for a task, and staying within the mid-point in a joint's range of motion.

Applying Ergonomic Principles

Lifting

Lifting anything applies the rule of ergonomics related to using the largest muscle group. The resource, erogonomics.org, refers to this as the "largest appropriate muscle group." You wouldn't use your forearm to push a light switch when an "appropriate" muscle is the one that operates the index finger. To lift heavier objects or move heavier items is where this principle is mainly concerned.

Most people are well aware that if you lift a heavy box by bending over and pulling up with the arms, your back will take the brunt of the weight, hence risk a tremendous injury to the back. That is why movers will wear thick belts. This harness supports the back and prevents it from doing the work. The largest muscles in the body are in the front thigh – the quadriceps. These should always take most of the weight and exertion when lifting. Here are some helpful tips when lifting:

- Bend down, not over. If you squat down, you must naturally use your legs to raise and lift the object with them.

- Work with a partner. Whenever possible, lighten the load by getting someone else to lift with you.

- Keep the back vertical. When the trunk is horizontal, it adds hundreds of pounds of pressure on just a tiny section of the spine that acts as a fulcrum, bearing most of the load.

- Keep objects you are lifting close to the body. The stress on the spine is exponentially related to the distance away from the object raised.

- When lifting a heavy object from above your head to lower it, get up close on a step stool to avoid holding the weight overhead with your arms. Again, closer is better when lifting.

Carrying Children

Many of the same principles that apply to lifting heavy objects apply to lifting and carrying children. You will often see an infant or toddler perched on a mother's hip. Think about her posture. Is her trunk vertical, or is it skewed to one side to compensate for the added weight on her hip?

There are many great devices to help make carrying children more manageable and safer. The best and safest choices allow the weight to be evenly distributed and keep the trunk and spine in good vertical alignment. A good example is an over-the-shoulder sling that holds an infant up to chest level in front of the parent. Do not use the sling for extended periods because the baby's weight gets to be very heavy. If this happens, the parent has to bend forward or backward to compensate for the added weight.

When carrying older or heavier children for any length of time, it is best to carry them on your back, piggyback style. A backpack carrier is suitable for walks or hikes because its waist straps distribute more weight to the hips than the back – again, using the larger muscles to carry the load.

When lifting a child out of a crib or playpen, get as close to the side as possible. If the sides of the crib lower, always do that first. This way, you will not have to lift above your waist, and it prevents awkward angles for your back. Wrap your arms around the child's midsection with one arm supporting their lower body, and bring them close to you before lifting upward. You may have to bend over to cradle an infant lying on his back, but you can still get him close to you before moving upward.

Standing up

When was the last time you thought about how you were getting out of bed in the morning or standing up from sitting in a chair? You probably never give it any thought unless it is uncomfortable or even painful. There are methods of standing up that relieve pain and prevent strain or injury to the back. Some of these apply the ergonomic principle of staying within the mid-range of joint motion.

Start the morning well by getting out of bed the correct way. Instead of springing up by arching the back and jumping to the floor, start by turning over into a side-lying position. Then swing your legs over the edge of the bed until they touch the floor and simultaneously press yourself up with your arms. From this seated position, then, you can use your thighs and arms together, if necessary, to push yourself to a standing position.

If you have the time, it is even better to do some simple stretching even before sitting up. You can extend your arms up over your head and, at the same time, push your legs out so your spine, arms, and legs all get a good stretch before being worked for the day.

When getting out of a chair, you can use the same steps as getting out of bed. If you are sunk deeply into a soft chair or sofa, scoot to the edge, so your feet are firmly planted on the floor before standing. This way, you are doing more pushing with your legs than swinging with your back for the additional momentum needed to get up from that sucked-in position.

Getting in and out of a car can also put a strain on the spine. We tend to get in by putting one leg in, swinging our back, twisting to a seated position, then bringing the other leg in. The same is true in reverse for getting out of the car. Instead, try going in backside first. It may look a little funny, but you can swivel both legs around simultaneously to face forward once you are seated. Getting out, you can swivel the whole torso and legs together until they are on the ground outside the car, then rise to a standing position.

Shoveling

Depending on how much dirt or snow you need to move, shoveling can lead to some major back problems. The problem is the weight of materials moved and the repetitive nature of the movement combined. Shoveling snow is a relatively common source of pain for those in northern climates. While this activity may not apply to everyone, its principles extend to yard work, construction, and basic chores.

Think about how you would dig a patch for your garden. Everyone uses one hand down low on the shovel handle and the dominant hand up at the top. We bend at the waist, pick up the load, and then twist and throw it someplace else. This mechanism is one of the easiest ways to injure your back! The combination of weight and twisting motion is a killer for backs.

Here are some better ways to make shoveling safer for your back:

- Bend at the knees to scoop up a small amount and throw it straight ahead instead of twisting to the side. Position yourself so that you don't have to turn to unload the weight.

- Shovel deep piles of snow or dirt in layers. Don't try to lift too much weight. It not only strains the back but can put severe stress on the heart.

- Change your grip on the shovel. By doing so, you will reduce the repetition to the same set of muscles and joints.

- Take time to stand up straight and rest. Give your back and arms a good stretch every few minutes.

Backpack Syndrome

You have, no doubt, seen small children going off to school with a backpack that goes from the top of their heads, clear down to the backs of their knees. You can only imagine what those poor children are carrying that might even match their body weight! Backpacks themselves are not bad. They are an excellent way to heft a substantial load. The back and hip muscles together are a strong group. The problem with backpacks, and even heavy satchels or briefcases, is how we carry them.

Whenever carrying a backpack, it is wise to use *both* shoulder straps. If there's a waist strap, use it. This feature helps distribute the weight from the back to the hips. If you must carry it on one shoulder to look "cool" or for convenience, then switch shoulders often. We can apply this logic to overloaded handbags and purses as well. Try to lighten the load whenever possible. Students carrying textbooks should opt to hold one or two books in their hands to balance the weight in their school bags.

Figure out what you really must take with you and what can stay at home, school, or the office. For briefcases, messenger-style bags, or satchels, you can put the strap over your head and across your chest to better distribute the weight. Carrying heavy bags on each side reduces strain on the back caused by compensating for more weight on one side of the body than the other.

The Alexander Technique

The Alexander Technique is a method of applying the principles of ergonomics that have stood the test of time. Today, people use this technique to help focus on their physical activities and become more conscious about moving, lifting, or simply standing.

This method of thinking about each movement trains the individual to observe and record their activities and posture, noting which may be harmful. From here, they can apply the three main rules of ergonomics to future movement. Its primary goal is to avoid, or at least reduce, the occurrence of repetitive stress injuries that are so common in today's workplace.

The history of the Alexander Technique dates back to long before the term ergonomics was commonplace. In the early 1900s, as the industrial revolution took a stronghold in the United States, factory workers on America's assembly lines were trained to be efficient. One worker doing the same task hour after hour and day after day was highly effective in producing large output for the factory owners. Enlightened owners, however, also recognized that injured workers did not produce as much. The Alexander Technique applied in these situations was probably the precursor to cross-training by moving people from one task to another. Not only did it ensure a worker was always available for any task, but it changed the physical strains on a single worker.

The Alexander Technique is still in use in virtually every profession, to some degree. Management consistently monitors work habits and makes changes to avoid repetitive stress injuries. Educating yourself with the Alexander Technique allows you to use the right amount of exertion with the right muscles for any task. It also tells you the appropriate amount of time before changing position or activity level.

Sleep Positions

We don't have much control over our sleep positions once we fall asleep. We move around in our sleep until our subconscious tells our body we are comfortable. The best way to ensure a good night's sleep, and a position that will promote a healthy and robust back, is to start advantageously.

The first step is to choose a mattress that supports good sleep. Personal preferences will be different from one person to the next. This is often a problem with couples trying to share a bed when they have different needs and preferences for mattress firmness. New styles of beds let you have different degrees of firmness on each side and make the movement and motion of the bedmate go nearly undetected.

The sleep position that you start in is unique to you. There is no right or wrong to this decision either. The spot you cozy into that might be most comfortable could depend on different biomechanical problems you have and what areas need extra care.

For example, if you have discomfort in your shoulder or upper back, you may find it more comfortable to lie on your side and sort of hug a pillow in your arms. This position relieves the pressure in the shoulder area by keeping the top shoulder propped up and unloaded. Likewise, hip pain reduces by placing a pillow between the knees.

Bent knees, while lying on your back, can alleviate lower back discomfort. You can hold this position passively with a pillow under the knees or by sleeping in a semi-reclined position in an adjustable bed or reclining chair.

Those who suffer from degenerative disc disease can often find comfort when sleeping on their stomachs. Stretching the spine like this opens the space between each vertebra, lessening pain and pressure on the disc area. Relieving the facet joints is the goal for these patients as well as those with osteoarthritis.

These simple changes in the way you go about everyday movement can promote a stronger, healthier back. Just always keep in mind the three basic laws of ergonomics: to change position often, use appropriate muscle groups, and don't overextend joints.

Chapter 16

Wellness and Prevention

It is much easier to prevent than to cure. Think about it. It is a no-brainer. If you can keep yourself healthy through diet, exercise, and controlling stress, you are much better off than dealing with the dis-ease or conditions created through poor choices.

Choosing to live a healthy lifestyle and care, not only for your spine but also for every part of the body and mind, should be a relatively simple choice. No one wants to be unhealthy. No one wants pain. No one wants to be limited in their movement or abilities, either physical or mental.

Sometimes it is only a matter of knowing what to do and how to do it. You know what you want the results to be, but you are unsure how to get from point A to B. This is where I come in. As a chiropractor, personally and professionally, I have committed to educating myself and others on how to get the most from their body and, in turn, get the most out of living a healthy, pain-free, and illness-free life.

Now, I am not saying that you will never get sick or injured if you consistently eat right, exercise, lift safely, and move properly. I *am* saying that you increase the likelihood that your body will be prepared to handle the external forces placed upon your body. With good nutrition and exercise, you naturally create a more robust immune system against toxins in the air, viruses brought on and spread by others. You are building a solid defense against a variety of diseases.

To protect yourself against injury, use regular exercise and a nutritious diet to build strong bones and muscles. An impact-related injury is now less likely to damage them. Likewise, a spine kept in alignment through preventative chiropractic care is easier to correct through a minor adjustment following an injury. Again, you sustain the spine blockage and restriction-free. The body can now keep itself healthy. Yes, an ounce of prevention is worth a pound of cure has never been more accurate than when it comes to your health and wellness.

Managing Stress

Far too little emphasis is placed today on the reality that emotional stress, mental trauma, and phobias can cause real and damaging physical reactions and responses in the body (see my rant on Fibromyalgia in the 'Conditions' chapter). When you are emotionally stressed, there are subtle changes in posture which strain the joints and muscles. These sometimes imperceptible changes leave them susceptible to injury. Mental stress can even cause compression in spinal joints, inflammation of nerves and muscles, and increased sensitivity in these areas.

There are many successful ways to reduce stress. One method may work perfectly for one person, while another person needs to try something different. Controlling stress is a highly individual process.

No two people go about it the same way. The key here is to find out what works for you and apply it whenever necessary.

There are some basic strategies to reduce stress. Within one of these, you will probably find a more specific method that works for you. The goal is to control the mind's stress with a mental or physical activity that brings about noticeable physical changes such as slowing the heart rate, lowering blood pressure, or releasing muscle tension. Any physical change brought about by mental stresses such as deadlines, work, or financial worries, can also be changed back to a more desirable state through stress-reduction techniques.

Stress Reducing Exercises

There are so many benefits to exercise, one of which is to reduce stress. Exercise does not have to entail a lengthy visit to the local gym or changing into a leotard and regimentally doing gymnastics. Exercise is simply moving in a way that gets the heart pumping and the blood flowing so that endorphins can release. Endorphins are those chemicals that make you feel a sense of joy and physical and mental wellness. Some people refer to it as a "natural high."

Here are some great exercises that require very little preparation and no equipment (okay, maybe some good shoes!) You can do them at a moment's notice to reduce stress and refresh both the mind and body.

- Take a brisk 20-minute walk in the sunshine
- Walk the dog at a slower pace for 30 minutes

- House and yard work. You need to do these chores anyway; why not use them to break up clusters of work at the computer to exercise large muscle groups and clear your mind?

Making time to reduce stress is equally as crucial as these spur-of-the-moment breaks. If you set aside a time each day to mentally and physically prepare yourself for the day or unwind at the end of a stressful day, you will have something to look forward to each day. I promise that if you make this time, it will be your period of renewal. It will become well-deserved "me time." You will come to protect it as a priority; you'll miss it when you don't take the time to de-stress. You will begin to see the benefits of prioritizing your health.

During this time you set aside for yourself, you can either exercise or engage in some other form of stress reduction. Here are some other great activities that require little skill or preparation:

- Meditation

- Tai Chi

- Yoga

- Stretching exercises

- Motivational or inspirational reading (remember it doesn't have to be physical. Nourishing the mind can reduce physical stress symptoms.)

Meditation

Meditation is a contributor to improving the function of the immune system. Studies conducted at the University of Wisconsin confirmed this fact. The study used a meditation technique called mindfulness-based stress reduction. Forty-eight healthy people were divided into two groups. They each received meditation training for eight weeks and also received a vaccine for influenza.

Evaluation of blood samples at the four and eight-week marks indicated increased antibodies at significant levels in the patients practicing the meditation techniques. This increase is a sure sign that the body's immune system is strong and healthy. Of even more importance is that a healthy immune system is central to enjoying overall good health.

There are meditation techniques you can use at any time and in any place. However, the most effective meditative practice to relieve mental and physical stress is when you can devote a specific amount of time to removing yourself from all external disruptions. It does not have to take up a lot of time, perhaps 10 to 20 minutes, but it should be a quiet time in a place where other people or the telephone cannot disturb you.

Mindfulness-Based Stress Reduction

The Mindfulness-Based Stress Reduction Technique (MBSR) for meditation was developed at the University of Massachusetts Medical Center in 1979. It is still widely practiced and regarded as effective today. Based on the ancient Buddhist technique of the same name – mindfulness – it proposes being aware of the present moment, every moment, without judgment.

Proponents of MBSR, after more than 20 years of research, have concluded that the results include everything from an increased ability to relax to improved self-esteem. They have also witnessed long-term reductions in physical and psychological symptoms.

The technique works by first increasing awareness in all aspects related to the individual. This awareness includes a sense of your physical being and mental self. It is based on the premise that we already have this knowledge of self within us but must bring it to the point of awareness.

MBSR helps with chronic pain or illness, headaches, high blood pressure, sleep, and anxiety disorders, among others. It also benefits those who have stresses related to work, home, or finances. These external stresses can also lead to the physical health problems listed.

The technique works by being mindful of surrounding sounds, including your breathing. It focuses on rhythm and patterns related to how we react to specific situations. Included in the technique are stretching exercises to come to a mindful and aware state of being.

Hypnosis & Mind-Body Technique

Hypnosis is not specifically a part of chiropractic but may have some merit in overall well-being. As it relates to health, the primary purpose of hypnosis is its ability to free the mind to change behaviors.

The basic theory is that if you can create positive thoughts, it will lead to positive actions. In between are positive feelings. To enjoy the best health, for example, you would use hypnosis to strengthen your mental focus on the concept that you are a healthy person. You would begin to feel healthy with those positive, focused thoughts. Feeling healthy in your mind would then allow you to be healthier in your body. The idea leads to reality, mind over matter.

People often misunderstand hypnosis. Just think of the silly portrayals of hypnotized people we have seen on television or in the movies. Hypnosis will not leave you vulnerable to someone making you get up and do the funky chicken dance before a crowd!

Hypnosis is not a state of sleep. Those who are under hypnosis are awake and aware of their surroundings. They can make conscious decisions while examining the unconscious. You will not do anything contrary to how you would want to behave in the situation.

You may better understand hypnosis by thinking of it as a highly focused concentration directed by a professional hypnotherapist. The hypnotherapist helps you to open a line of communication between the conscious and subconscious minds. Our subconscious mind is gathering and storing information from all around us and holds that information. It is helpful to us when a reactive type of response is needed.

Logical thinking of the conscious mind is not always aware of the contents of the subconscious database. That is where hypnosis comes into play. When memories and other information from the subconscious mind become available to the conscious mind, this information can improve behavior, change a habit, or release us from mental stresses we may not have even been aware we had. These unconscious, mental stresses can be contributing to real physical health problems.

Acupuncture

This ancient Chinese method of inserting fine needles into the body to induce a physiological response is more than 4,000 years old. It relates directly to the idea of many other alternative medicines, including chiropractic, that the body has energy running through it. In Chinese, the energy is referred to as Qi and is pronounced "chee." Qi has a direct impact on the balance and wellness of all systems in the body.

Just like with nerve signals, Qi can have interference that prevents optimal health. The acupuncturist aims to remove the obstacles, just like the chiropractor removes the restriction in the spine. Perhaps that is why many chiropractors also incorporate acupuncture or the non-invasive, more massage-like form, acupressure, into their practices.

Acupuncture also has a body map with specific stimulus points related to organs and systems in the body. Sometimes acupuncture needles are inserted with a small electrical impulse added to stimulate the area further and remove the interference.

According to acupuncture philosophy, energy flows down pathways called meridians. The meridians need to be free from interference or obstructions – or stagnation in acupuncture terminology – and must stay in balance to achieve optimal health.

Tai Chi

Tai Chi is all about balance and harmony in the body. It goes very well with the chiropractic way of health care, as both strive for that balance.

The balanced state within Tai Chi is often referred to as Yin & Yang. The premise behind both Tai Chi and Chinese medicine is to increase the natural energy in the body. In chiropractic philosophy, we refer to that natural energy as innate intelligence. When Qi is not flowing correctly in the body, there is a feeling of not being well. Conversely, a free-flowing Qi within oneself leads to a sense of well-being.

Tai Chi can be considered both a physical and mental exercise. Specific movements and positions awaken or release energy flow. Breathing techniques and exercises go hand in hand with these movements. These form sets and activities have different purposes, but all improve muscle tone, balance, flexibility, mobility, and work to improve concentration - all through releasing greater energy flow.

Tai Chi can be done at home with videos to guide you. More and more classes and schools specific to the Chinese method are also popping up as people become more knowledgeable. Its value has been recognized globally, and has become more accepted as a viable method of maintaining good health.

Yoga

It is only fitting that we discuss yoga in this chapter, although many of you reading this have a deep understanding and exposure to it already. India is the birthplace of yoga practice and had very religious Hindu connotations in its earliest iterations. Yoga has many different applications for good health. There are specific movements, called poses or asanas, which can help with blood pressure, insomnia, osteoporosis, and stress. There are dozens of poses known to help with even more ailments and the prevention of them.

To perform yoga, the only "equipment" you need is an open mind and perhaps a good foam mat. The mat helps make some of the poses more comfortable. Loose clothing won't restrict your movements and will help in the practice. There are several poses in Yoga explicitly designed for stress reduction. The following is a list of poses with the common English name.

Stress Reducing Yoga Poses

Pose	Purpose/Benefit
Salutation Seal	Induces a state of meditation
Child's Pose	Suitable for returning to a restful, balanced state between other movements

Bharadvaja's Twist	Serves as a "tonic" to cleanse the abdominal organs and nourish the spine

Cobra Pose	Helps with spinal flexibility and opens the chest
Plow Pose	Used to reduce backache and promotes sound sleep
Noose Pose	Good for releasing tension
Supported Headstand	Has a calming effect on the brain and strengthens the whole body
Corpse Pose	Achieves a state of total relaxation
Bridge Pose	Rejuvenates tired legs
Standing Forward Bend	Soothes the mind and stretches the hamstrings
Extended Triangle Pose	Standing pose to center yourself.

Each pose in yoga can be challenging to achieve the first few times you try it. It may seem like so much effort is hardly capable of reducing stress. Just trying to clasp your hands behind your back might create more stress than it relieves! Rest assured, each yoga pose is achievable. With every session, there will be more and more flexibility and ease in completing the pose. As this happens, more of your mind can get away from the movement and the strain it seems to cause at first. Sticking with the program, in just a few short weeks, you will be able to realize its great stress-reducing benefits.

Yoga is commonly prescribed in India as a means of injury rehabilitation. It is vital that you use caution, perform the movements slowly and carefully, and do not ignore any exacerbation of pain. As wonderful and ancient of an art form yoga is, it's not the "be all, end all" of human performance and rehabilitation. I've seen several avid yogis who strain too hard during their sessions and create injuries from their practice. Chiropractic care can help attain deeper poses, increased range of motion, and improve your practice's depth. The teaching method should also match your injury, so having an instructor with knowledge of common ailments would be beneficial for your recovery.

Chapter 17

The Mistakes We Make Everyday

Each new day we make unconscious mistakes that are putting our spinal health and overall wellness at risk. You can find some of the most common ones here, as well as a method to correct or avoid making the same mistakes day after day.

From morning to night, there are slight modifications we can make to improve posture and protect our backs. These tips include all of the principles of ergonomics. They show subtle and straightforward ways we can reduce the tension that leads to stress on the back. Some of these you may already subscribe to; that's a great start. Some of these might be extremely obvious, which is also a good thing. We just want to cover all our bases and make sure the basics are down pat!

- Start the day off right with a good stretch. Hug your knees to your chest, individually, then together. While holding both knees in, roll gently to each side.

- When brushing your teeth, don't hunch over the sink. Stand up straight and bend at the waist, pushing your hips backward when you need to rinse.

- Make sure chairs are the right height and depth for your body. You should sit back and still have 2 inches between the end of the chair and the back of your knees. This seated position will help you hold a good posture and prevent knee pain.

- Ensure that you have adequate lighting for all tasks. One of the leading causes of tension headaches is poor lighting and the eye strain that results.

- Avoid wearing high-heeled shoes too often. They can cause spinal stress because the weight distributes unevenly between heel and toe. Alternatively, change into your heels only when required.

- Sitting with your legs crossed is a big no-no and can eventually lead to spinal misalignment. Ideally, you should sit with both feet on the floor.

- Holding a telephone tucked between your shoulder and neck can cause the joints to lock up in the upper back, neck, and shoulders. Use your hand or a headset if you need to have your hands free.

- If you have a desk job, be sure to get up and move around frequently. It is important to change positions often, especially if you are making repetitive motions while sitting, such as typing at a computer. My recommendation is to stand every 25-30 minutes and do something else for 1-5 minutes.

- Find ways to reduce emotional stress and tension. That will carry into your posture if left unattended. Meditation does wonders, but don't take my word for it; explore the many free and paid apps available on your smartphone. If you're new to meditation, there are guides in abundance to help you get started.

- Get plenty of sleep on a quality mattress and a good pillow that supports the neck and spine.

Chapter 18

Chiropractic for Life

Chiropractic is a lifelong plan for wellness. Every stage of life can benefit from routine chiropractic care. Chiropractic is helpful for infants, children, adolescents, young adults, middle-aged, and seniors. It is for those who are generally in good health and those who suffer from specific conditions.

Because the body has its own ability to heal, it knows what condition it should be in and how to keep itself healthy. And so chiropractic, which keeps this ability in good working condition, should be for everyone. Unlike a medical doctor you may see once a year for a checkup, chiropractic should be part of a preventative health care routine. If this routine incorporates into your wellness plan, it can help you stay healthier and get more out of life.

The human body is a miraculous entity. It can perform functions when we don't even realize it is working. It's on the job 24/7. You still breathe in your sleep, and the heart keeps on beating. It does all of this without you having to lift a finger; it even regulates itself to accommodate changes we force upon it. For example, when we run, the body automatically speeds up the heart rate and quickens our breathing. Hence, the extra needed oxygen is available and transported to the muscles to do extra work.

Chiropractic plays a vital role in allowing this system to do its job correctly. When spinal restrictions occur, those blockages that reduce the messages transmitted by the nerve, then the body's ability to correct what might be wrong are hindered. Regular, preventative chiropractic care will allow a free flow of signals to the whole body.

Each stage of life brings with it a different set of potential health problems and ailments. That is why even the 2-hour-old newborn infant can benefit from the gentle touch of a chiropractor to ensure the rigors of the birthing process did not cause any vertebrae to become misaligned.

`Chiropractic for Infants and Children*

Childhood illnesses such as ear infections, asthma, food allergies, and even Attention Deficit Disorder (ADD) are becoming so commonplace that new parents often accept them as simply part of childhood. The chiropractic way of thinking is that the creation of human life does not automatically come with built-in problems and illnesses. It is complete and perfect until external factors change that. That is not to discount the fact that genetic factors or environmental hazards can impact the life of an ideal human being's health.

Now, healthy babies are born every day, and many of them have no issues at all and never receive chiropractic care. Many of you have never been to a chiropractor, and you turned out fine, right? It's true; the average healthy baby is born well and can stay well, even in a world of common childhood illnesses. But what if the body is allowed to communicate messages freely to keep this perfect baby as healthy as the day it was born?

Six Facts That Will Keep Children Healthy

Want a healthier child? There are six facts about chiropractic that will keep children healthy if you choose to understand them, abide by them, and implement their meaning. By understanding these six facts, you will have the tools to remove most of the interferences that make people, especially children, unhealthy.

FACT #1:

The nervous system controls the functioning of every cell in the body and especially the immune system. Keeping the spine in perfect order can boost the immune system's strength by 200 to 400 percent.

FACT #2:

You can eliminate childhood health problems by having your child examined by an expert who knows what to look for and what questions to ask about bumps, falls, and normal childhood activities. An examination of the spine regularly by a qualified chiropractor will help the doctor know if anything has changed. Corrections made accurately immediately open up the way for optimal nerve signals to pass through the entire body.

FACT #3:

You indeed are what you eat. Nutrition is the secret to creating a strong immune system, and children must eat a variety of healthy foods rich in vitamins and minerals. Sometimes supplements are used to make up for shortcomings, but they should not be the primary source of nutrients.

FACT #4:

You need to identify problems as they arise to fix them in time. Routine examinations of your child's spine will ensure that restrictions are corrected before significant issues can arise.

FACT #5:

Adjustments are needed to keep the body working at 100 percent of its capacity. Your brain must not have interference when trying to communicate with and organize the body's other systems.

FACT # 6:

Be consistent. It is the key not only in parenting or disciplining children but in keeping them healthy. Start early and continue with proper chiropractic care.

The following section discusses chiropractic and its role in treating the most common ailments associated with children.

Chiropractic for Ear Infections

Ear infections are just a normal part of early childhood, right? Wrong! Ear infections, technically known as *otitis media*, are an infection of the inner ear. While it is common to get an ear infection during childhood, it does not have to become a chronic childhood condition.

Most young children before the age of 2 will have at least one ear infection. There are more than 10 million new cases every year of ear infections. They account for 35% of all visits to the pediatrician. An ear infection is no small matter, yet it is not the grounds for surgery that mainstream pediatrics routinely suggests.

Either viral or bacterial infections cause middle ear infections. They most often occur because of a build-up of fluid in the eardrum. When the fluid can't drain, infections can occur. The objective then should be to get rid of the goo and avoid the condition. The medical field does this through surgery. The insertion of ear tubes intends to open the canal and allow fluid to drain. The number one surgery for children under two is for the insertion of ear tubes.

There are several problems with this method of treatment. One is that it doesn't always provide lasting treatment. Between 20% and 30% of children receiving ear tubes have to have the procedure repeated. The insertion of ear tubes usually requires the usage of general anesthesia; some of these kids have to have it done for yet a second time.

Even if a child doesn't undergo surgery, the mainstream method of treating ear infections does little to help the child in the long run. The primary non-surgical treatment is antibiotics. While this may treat a bacterial infection, it does nothing for a viral infection. It sets the child up for more infections in the future because it allows common pathogens time to become resistant to the antibiotics. Antibiotics also do nothing to improve drainage.

Chiropractic can both alleviate a child's painful symptoms of the ear infection and deal with the cause. The fluid buildup due to poor drainage is what allows infections to form. If the ear canal can open in a non-surgical manner, isn't that what is best for the child?

Chiropractic can open the ear canal and aid drainage of the eardrum by manipulating C1, or the first cervical vertebra in the spine. This method used by the renowned chiropractor, Dr. Joan Fallon, was very effective. She discovered that with frequent adjustments over six months, her young patient's bodies drained excess fluid well. The result was an absence of ear infections.

If the child did experience an ear infection, it gave the body the information it needed to fight off future infections. By not stifling the body's own natural responses and ensuring there was no blockage of the nerves in the upper cervical spine, the children under her care got fewer ear infections.

Chiropractic in the Treatment of Asthma

Asthma, in adults and children, is on the rise. Scientists, allergists, and other doctors are not exactly sure why. Asthma has always been primarily a genetic condition where the airways become restricted because of muscle hyper-responsiveness. However, according to the World Health Organization, between 100 and 150 million people worldwide are being treated for asthma today. This astonishing statistic can't all be from hereditary issues! There are environmental factors that have led to the increase in asthma, mainly amongst children.

Much of the rise in asthma is environmental. Modern manufacturing produces more allergens, and more of them stay trapped in our homes and offices because of improved construction and insulation methods. This current process is why there are more cases of asthma in industrialized nations.

Asthma is usually treated with medication. The medications found in inhalers intend to open the small bronchial passages in the lungs and allow for better airflow. The medicines are steroid-type drugs, specifically corticosteroids. Do we want our children to be inhaling steroids? Most parents would prefer a less invasive way to help their children breathe easier.

There are many side effects of the use of inhaled steroids. Most children experience inhibited growth in the first year that they inhale the drug, although they eventually return to a typical growth pattern. Other side effects are more long-term and show up later in life, including osteoporosis, hypertension, and diabetes - all severe conditions.

Chiropractic has successfully been used to treat both adults and children with asthma. There is no cure for asthma, but the treatments are effective and can provide comfortable relief. Acute asthma attacks may still require an inhaler, but it would be better if prevented altogether. That is the purpose behind chiropractic in treating asthma – to prevent asthma attacks in the first place.

Some methods in preventing asthma attacks are very proactive wellness techniques that go hand in hand with the chiropractic philosophy. These include an excellent nutritional base for children. When the immune system is functioning well, and the body is well-equipped with the proper nutrients, it can correct many factors that may trigger an asthma attack.

Secondly, exercise is a beneficial factor in preventing asthma attacks for those who often suffer attacks from exertion. It seems counterintuitive at first; exertion brings on asthma, but you want me to exert myself? Here's the logic: in a sense, the child prepares their body to handle the attack by conditioning the lungs. Again, the proactive approach is preventative in nature. Instead of allowing the lungs to languish in a weak state, you can fight against the possibility of an attack by gradually increasing the lung's workload.

The goal of chiropractic in treating a child with asthma is to prevent attacks *and* improve the child's overall quality of life. A child who must limit their participation in normal childhood activities will not be as happy, even if that means no asthma attacks. The goal with chiropractic is to improve both the quality and quantity of activities in which the child can participate while preventing asthma attacks.

Chiropractic is in its infancy in the treatment of childhood asthma. There are no conclusive studies to date that prove chiropractic can prevent attacks. In most practices that treat children with asthma, chiropractors hypothesize a release of endorphins or other internal reactions caused by spinal manipulation help with pulmonary function. Chiropractic is to be used with traditional medications until more conclusive research exists about its effect on asthma. One fact that has definitive proof is that children who regularly visit the chiropractor can improve posture, including the mechanical function and structure of the ribs and shoulders encasing the lungs. Removing any physical restrictions of breathing allows children (and parents!) to breathe easier.

Chiropractic Treatment for Food Allergies

Getting rid of the symptoms from food allergies can be one of the easiest, most controllable treatments or one of the most challenging. Clearly, if you know what you ate that brought on the allergic reaction, you can eliminate it from your diet. The challenge lies in uncovering what you're allergic to if it's not immediately apparent.

Allergy testing for food allergies is often done by injecting small amounts of the suspected allergen into the skin and observing the result. The substance that causes redness or swelling is the culprit. To treat the allergy, simply remove the food from the diet. Problem solved.

When the allergen cannot be isolated, it, therefore, cannot be removed. With infants just starting on solid foods, parents introduce only one food at a time for several days to make sure the baby doesn't experience any rashes, vomiting, or diarrhea. If all is well, then a new food is introduced. This method allows parents to see which foods are agreeable with the baby's tender system.

Chiropractic takes a similar approach in treating food allergies, or any other allergies for that matter. Balancing the nervous system, which is the underlying treatment in every condition, allows the body to fight off allergies – food or otherwise. Improving the nervous system's function improves the immune system and its histamine response defense system. It is an indirect observation that chiropractic treats the allergy, and as always, there's still more research to do.

A lifestyle where stress is under control is one in which fewer allergies will appear. Stress increases cortisol production and taxes the adrenal glands. This makes the body susceptible to allergies. Trying to avoid foods laden with chemicals and additives also prevents food allergies. The chiropractic way of life focuses on eating whole, preferably organic foods, which the body can use for good nutrition and health.

Managing ADD through Chiropractic

Attention Deficit Disorder (ADD) and Attention Deficit Hyperactivity Disorder (ADHD) diagnoses are increasing rapidly. Are there really more cases? Or is it more likely that schools and doctors are snapping this one-size-fits-all label on any child who is active, bored, learns differently, or is experiencing some kind of stress at home or school? These are conditions that professionals often misdiagnose as ADD or ADHD.

In reality, ADD and ADHD have accompanying symptoms that go far beyond being unable to sit through a classroom storytime or showing some kind of aggressive behavior. Those who are genuinely afflicted with the disorder usually also experience other symptoms such as sensitivity to light, sound, and touch. They may also experience tics or tremors and have obvious postural problems. This last symptom is one that chiropractic best addresses. It may also be the symptom that, when treated, alleviates many of the others.

Doctors of Chiropractic and, more specifically, Chiropractic Neurologists are involved in the impact the postural muscles have on brain activity. When there is a musculoskeletal imbalance, there will be an imbalance in brain activity. This imbalance results in the uneven development of the brain, with one side outpacing the other. Theoretically, this is the underlying condition associated with children who truly have ADD or ADHD.

Brain stimulation is the primary method that chiropractors employ in accelerating the development of the lagging side of the brain. Incredible results are achieved through a series of tests that stimulate auditory and visual functions within the brain. Several examples of these tests include: a flashing light, blocking light with special glasses, or listening to music with just one ear. These therapies go on for a period of only a few months before noticing measurable results.

Improving the under-functioning area of the brain is only one step chiropractors take in treating children with ADD. They also recommend lifestyle changes that promote better nutrition and avoid unnatural ingredients such as dyes and preservatives. This helps regulate biochemical imbalances that may also contribute to the child's ADD symptoms by improving the diet in general and creating a healthier balance.

Improving a child's specific musculoskeletal imbalances and nutrition works together to treat ADD and ADHD without the use of other medications. Although medications are effective when used, they stop working once the drug is discontinued, which creates an undesirable dependence into adulthood. With chiropractic methods, the change is permanent because the brain is stimulated and allowed to develop properly.

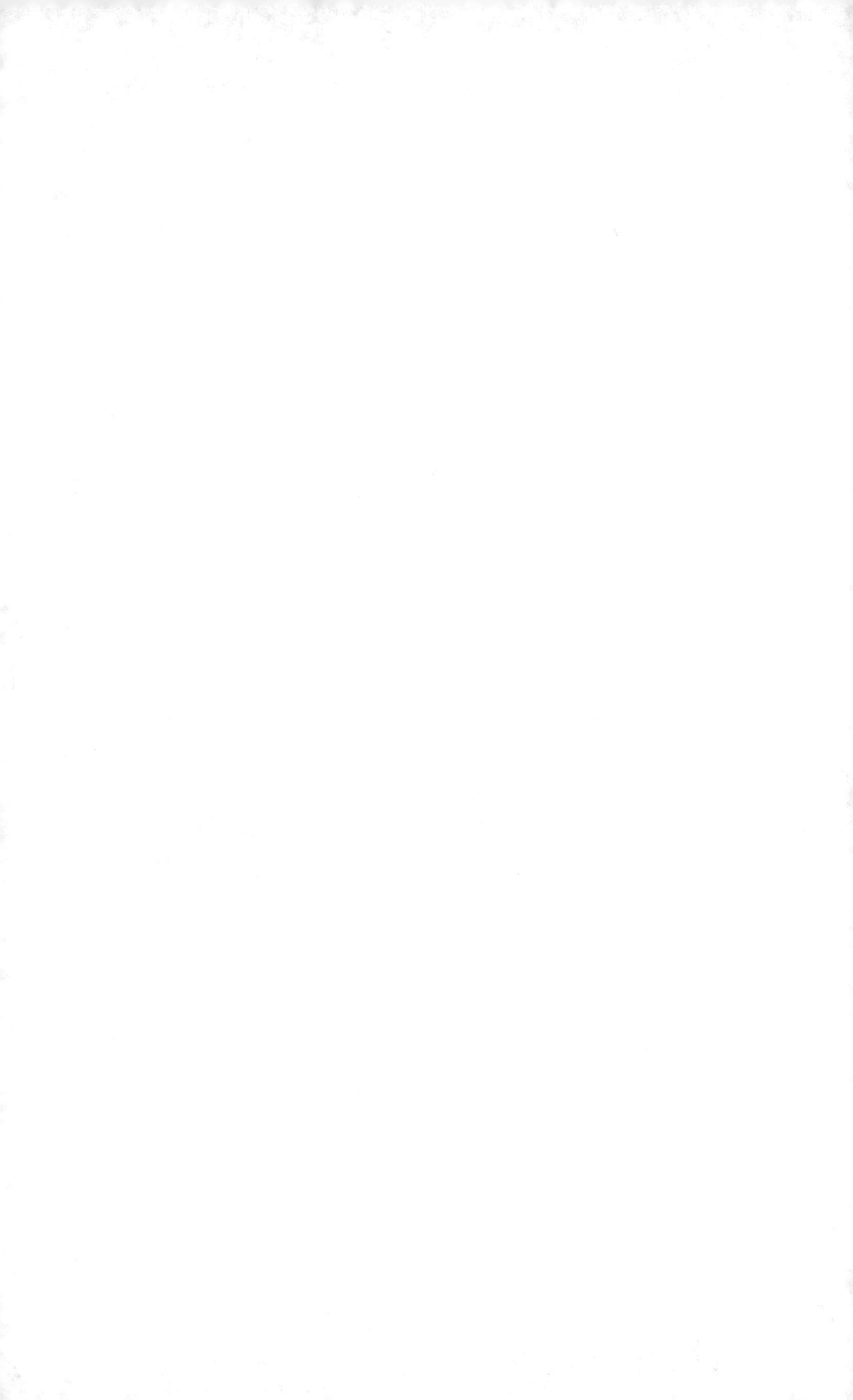

9 798541 332124